IT IS WELL WITH MY SOUL

CHURCHES AND INSTITUTIONS
COLLABORATING FOR PUBLIC HEALTH

REVEREND MELVIN TUGGLE

⅃ PUBLIC HEALTH ASSOCIATION
ⅢNGTON, DC

It Is Well With My Soul

Churches and Institutions
Collaborating for Public Health

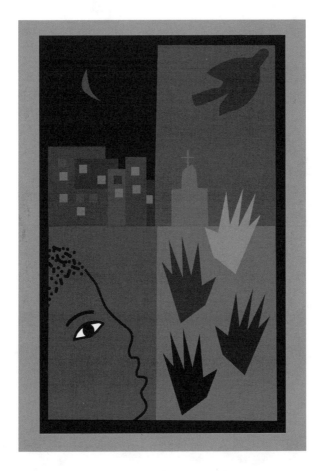

Reverend Melvin Tuggle

American Public Health Association
Washington, DC

American Public Health Association
800 I Street, NW
Washington, DC 20001

Mohammad N. Akhter, MD, MPH
Executive Director

Printed and bound in the United States of America

Cover Design: Adjoa J. Burrowes

Typesetting: Ruth Burke for Magnificent Publications, Inc.

Set in: Garamond

Printing and Binding: Kirby Lithographic

ISBN: 0-87553-180-6

1.5M 8/00

Library of Congress card catalog number 00-106868

APHA Mission Statement

The American Public Health Association is an association of individuals and organizations working to improve the public's health. It promotes the scientific and professional foundation of public health practice and policy, advocates the conditions for a healthy global society, emphasizes prevention, and enhances the ability of members to promote and protect environmental and community health.

Table of Contents

About the Author

D<small>R. MELVIN BAXTER TUGGLE II</small>, Pastor of the (Beautiful) Garden of Prayer Baptist Church in Baltimore, Maryland, initiated the formation of the partnership between Johns Hopkins University, the W.K. Kellogg Foundation, and the East Baltimore Church and Neighborhood Communities. He is also the past president of the Clergy United for the 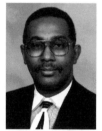 Renewal of East Baltimore, Inc. (CURE), representing 268 ecumenical churches, and the founder and president of Heart, Body, and Soul, Inc., the health initiative of CURE.

Reverend Tuggle has appointments in the School of Public Health and Hygiene, the School of Medicine, and the School of Nursing at Johns Hopkins University and has taught classes in the following courses: Tobacco Control: A Public Health Perspective; Careers and Issues in Public Health; Cardiovascular Epidemiology; and Community Health. He has traveled on behalf of the East Baltimore Community and Johns Hopkins to five model leadership development conferences conducted by the W.K. Kellogg Foundation to encourage a combination of academic and realistic community public health issues and solutions.

Tuggle has served as a national consultant for tobacco control in urban populations for the National Lung Association. He has presented speeches and seminars for the National Institutes of Health, the Congress of Black Churches, the American Heart Association, the National Minority Health Association, the Centers for Disease Control and Prevention, Meharry Medical Center, and the National Minority Nursing Conference, among others.

This active pastor developed and implemented a program that for the first two years of operation provided services to more than 4,000 high-risk persons. He has shared expertise with many national groups, has been interviewed on numerous radio talk shows, has been featured in newspaper and magazine articles, and has appeared on television. Tuggle's work has attracted the attention of media, church, and medical representatives throughout and beyond the United States. His previous publications include "A Partnership with Minority Populations: A Community Model of Effectiveness Research," "The Heart, Body, and Soul Program: Churches as a Way to Lower Heart Disease Risk," and "Community-Derived Cardiovascular Risk Reduction in Urban African-American Churches."

Reverend Dr. Tuggle firmly believes that if he can help someone as he travels life's journey, then his living will not be in vain.

Foreword

NOWHERE ARE THE NATIONAL ISSUES concerning health care more magnified than in urban underserved minority communities, which suffer significantly higher rates of premature morbidity, disability, and mortality than the rest of the population. Many of the causes of this disparity—such as smoking, hypertension, diabetes, substance abuse, violence, vision problems, obesity, and various cancers—are either preventable or treatable and controllable. Whatever emerges from national health care system reform, it will be insufficient if significant progress is not made in decreasing the gap in the health and functional status of underserved minority populations.

In this book, Reverend Melvin Tuggle addresses these issues directly and provides both understanding of the factors that have precipitated this crisis and new approaches to address and solve these problems. Applying the experiences of African Americans, the most populous underserved minority group, Reverend Tuggle provides a comprehensive, innovative, and practical approach to addressing contemporary public health problems from a community-based perspective. He weaves together his experience and expertise as a pastor, community leader, and pioneer to provide clear guidance for the development of effective, sustainable programs to enhance the health and functional status of the African American community.

Reverend Tuggle displays for us the crucial role of the church in the African American population and shows how churches and other public and private institutions (for example, academic health centers, health departments, schools, community groups, foundations, and national health institutes) can develop true partnerships to enhance the public health of African Americans. From his own personal experience, he describes the challenges, as well as the opportunities to collaborate for change, in enhancing the availability, accessibility, and quality of programs to promote health and prevent and control disease. Others will benefit from the clear principles and lessons that the author provides in his discussion of the criteria for developing successful community-based partnership programs anywhere, as partnership development; the role and training of community health workers; leadership development; disseminating the program; funding and securing funding; and planning for sustainability. In these principles, Reverend Tuggle offers guidance that will be invaluable to church, community, and institutional leaders, as well as community residents.

Reverend Tuggle has brought together, for us, all the crucial elements for a serious response to our national health crisis, and in particular the continuing, unacceptable poor health status of underserved and minority populations. In this vein, he has performed a public service. This book should be welcomed by and essential reading for leaders and students alike in the church, the community, local, state, and national government, and the health professions.

David M. Levine MD, ScD, MPN
Associate Director of Medicine
Johns Hopkins University Medical School

Preface

Effective interaction with inner-city populations is dependent upon the use of models, strategies, and techniques that have been successful in inner-city areas. Importing programs that worked in rural, suburban, and middle-to-upper class communities will not work. Each environment presents its own culture, challenges, and forms of communication, and recognizing and understanding these are paramount to the success of any public service program.

In this book, we concentrate on inner cities and the specific challenges faced when working in these communities, home to millions of our nation's population. Within these neighborhoods are high incidences of disease and death from preventable illnesses. You may ask why. The reasons include poorly built houses, clustered close together and generally in undesirable environmentally degraded areas. Crowded conditions contribute to the spread of viruses, germs, and contagious diseases. City sewers clog and are not attended for weeks, if at all. Minimal trash removal is common, resulting in overflows that usually end up on the ground around a dumpster or in an empty lot. Most of the housing units do not have adequate plumbing and heating systems, or else the residents simply cannot afford adequate services. Meals are planned based on what is cheap and what is going to stretch far enough to last several days and fill stomachs, rather than on nutritional value. The few inner-city grocery stores often offer substandard products and too many prepared and processed items. In a survival mode, they have to choose between buying food, paying rent, taking care of the water and heat bill, and other basic needs. Unfortunately, health care is often at the bottom of the list, if on the list at all.

I know this sounds depressing, but it really is right here in the United States. Not just in one or two communities or in particular regions, but throughout the country. Don't be discouraged, though, because change can occur, not through one person perhaps but certainly through partnerships. In my community of East Baltimore, site of the world-renowned Johns Hopkins Hospital, people were dying at an alarming rate. How could that be when one of the greatest medical institutions in the United States was within walking distance of these residents?

It's simple: there was no connection or relationship between the hospital and the community. They did not understand each other and frankly were intimidated and afraid of each other. Realizing this, the community, and particularly the church, began to talk and interact with the hospital and foundations. The group addressed issues head-on, sometimes butting heads. However, everyone pulled together to form and start a highly successful plan to save lives and money.

The first and perhaps biggest challenge is self-reflection, to better understand the reasons for fear, misconceptions, misinformation, biases, and prejudices. Left unresolved, these factors will inhibit the success of any program. A sincere commitment must be made to changing the way things are viewed. Key issues are understanding cultural differences between whites and African Americans, acknowledging the reluctance of African Americans to trust whites, seeing everyone as equal but perhaps with different experiences and purposes, and above all, working through the communication channels that are unique to African American communities.

Having considered all there is to unlearn and learn, one may think that interacting effectively with African Americans, or any other ethnic group, is nearly impossible. Untrue! The key is to learn how the particular ethnic group and community operate. Learning this takes a lot of groundwork, most effectively on sacred ground: the churches within the community. The churches must be involved with any effort to initiate and start effective inner-city public health programs. With the church, expect acceptance, access, information, support, and above all a level of trust. Without the involvement of the church, programs may be delayed or even stopped altogether.

On the other side, the church needs the resources of the institutions, foundations, and hospitals. Without those resources, whether it is educational materials, community health workers, or screening programs, the church remains somewhat powerless to deal with the medical and technical needs of the community. In short, partnering is essential for success and it takes work "on both sides of the fence." This book will be instructive for institutions and community groups alike. It provides a base of knowledge on how both "sides" operate, what both expect, and the best way of interacting with each other.

It Is Well With My Soul has been developed for use as a stand-alone study and reference guide, a training text, and a general resource for anyone involved or seeking to become involved in partnering for effective inner-city public health. I hope that its contents will help you establish and maintain the relationships that are necessary for inner-city residents and institutions to benefit from what both can offer today and tomorrow.

CHAPTER ONE

Churches, Cities, & Challenges

The Beginning of the Black Church

UNDERSTANDING AND REMEMBERING the early history of the black church gives all partners a greater sense and base from which to leverage its power and influence. Now deeply rooted in the concrete of inner cities where nothing else seems to thrive, the black church sprouted first in the soil of the South where cotton and tobacco grew, in the rocky red clay of the mountains where mining provided valuable coal, or any place where blacks, many as slaves, lived. These roots extend from the church to the minds and hearts of most African Americans whether or not they are "churched." Although unspoken, there is an almost inborn respect and reverence for the black church and its leaders. And many past and present African American leaders have been or are still practicing ministers; for example, Reverend Francis Cardozo, elected Secretary of State of South Carolina in 1868, and more familiar names such as Reverend Adam Clayton Powell, Reverend Dr. Martin Luther King Jr., Reverend Jesse Jackson, and Reverend Floyd Flake, U.S. Representative from New York.

The connection between churches, ministers, and politics dates from slavery, through the evolution of the independence of blacks, and the civil rights movement. Although many would say they still are not free and do not have civil rights today, that is another story. Although whites and blacks worshiped together in the 1700s, the blacks (mostly slaves) never had real freedom or equality in the church, nor were they able to select their own religion. Just as buses and water fountains were to be segregated, so were the early church pews. The story often left untold is that of the earliest black churches, when groups of slaves gathered in the dark woods or in safehouses, the only places where slaves could socialize, pray, seek help, and express what they had to keep hidden from their masters.

During the "Great Awakening" in the 1740s, these informal services of black slaves were welcomed with both enthusiasm and fear. The clandestine services were held at great risk, as slaves were allowed to attend only churches pastored by white ministers. Yet they supported the spiritual and emotional needs of the slaves; there they could shout, sing, and comfort each other. Whites considered these unsupervised meetings a threat. By the "Second Awakening" in 1780, revival meetings, still usually held in the woods and in tents, had begun to sweep across the country. Attracting large numbers of people, who gathered to sing spirituals and shout aloud what they were feeling, these revivals also heightened the fear among whites of black churches and congregationalism. Lynchings, threats, prohibitions, and church burnings continued throughout the years, perhaps because whites thought that the revivalists were plotting to harm them? Without a doubt, there is power when people of like minds and purposes of any race come together. However, the black church has never in its history served to attack, harm, or destroy anyone. Its importance lies in its positive and peaceful accomplishments.

The established black church in America dates back at least as early as 1608. Records show that several freed slaves in a settlement near St. Augustine, Florida, became Christians, and that in 1623 a young son of free blacks in Jamestown, Virginia, was the first to be baptized in the English colonies. While historians have debated the exact date and place of the first black Baptist congregation in America, there is general agreement that it began between 1750 and 1775 in Silver Bluff, South Carolina. A slave named George Liele and a white preacher traveled along the Savannah River preaching to other slaves and ultimately established a church of free blacks and slaves. Other churches grew out of the secret congregations of slaves that continued to meet in those places where they were unseen and felt safe.

Pioneers of Social Service

The slaves who started the black church were pioneers of what we now call organizations, advisors, counselors, and social service providers. At these early churches, slaves could find advice, food, clothing, information, and more; later, the churches developed more formal methods of providing assistance. These early, makeshift churches mark somewhat of an evolution of the church, as slaves stopped attending racially mixed churches with white leadership, then moved to separate churches still under white leadership, and eventually established black churches with black leaders. The latter congregational makeup is what we see most often today. Churches are among the most segregated institutions in the country, largely because of their origins and history.

Free blacks and slaves migrated in great numbers from the South to other areas, especially to what are now northern inner cities. They brought the independent black church movement with them so they could worship with dignity and freedom in their own special style. The church also continued its tradition of being a service provider by hiding escaped slaves, housing newcomers, and offering a meal or two. For many blacks, the ministers were the only ones who made a conscious and consistent effort to help and to rally others to do the same. They also spoke the word of God freely, and sometimes loudly, to people more accustomed to quiet whispers. The church and its leaders represented long-sought freedom, and ministers were among the most respected and visible in the community, in many cases the only positive role models. Churches served as multipurpose buildings and were often the only place where blacks felt accepted and comfortable. In all areas, not just inner cities, churches were also schools, recreation centers, and funeral homes. Much later, churches were the sites for free food distribution, Head Start programs, health tests, and more. When some of these social service programs ended or moved, the church assumed the responsibility of providing these services to a growing and needy community.

These changes confirmed the community's dependence on the church, dating back to its beginning. The Acts of the Apostles, 2:45-47, shows how believers devoted themselves to giving to everyone as they had a need, sharing food and their homes gladly and sincerely. For the church, serving the needs of others is a mandate from God as depicted in Matthew, 25:35-36/40: "For I was hungry and you gave me something to eat, I was thirsty and you gave me something to drink, I was a stranger and you invited me in, I needed clothes and you clothed me, I was sick and you looked after me, I was in prison and you came to visit me... I tell you the truth, whatever you did for one of the least of these brothers of mine, you did for me." To be obedient to God, the church is responsible for those in need and must lift the least. As Reverend Dr. Martin Luther King Jr. stated: "Any religion that professes to be concerned with the souls of [people] and is not concerned about the slums that damn them, the economic conditions that strangle them, and the social conditions that cripple them is a spiritually moribund religion awaiting burial." In essence, churches have no choice.

Cities and the Great Exodus

Colored, Negro, Black, and now African American communities— the names used to describe Americans of African descent have changed along with the community. For freed slaves living in the South, the community meant living with relatives and friends, sometimes two or three families in one dwelling. Everything needed was found nearby. All activities took place in the community. There was still a fear of the white man and self-righteous, convicting groups such as the Ku Klux Klan. Communities began to change as blacks moved out, searching for better employment, education, and simply to see another part of the United States. Some of them came back to teach or to operate businesses; however, most moved permanently, particularly to growing cities. In these cities, they could be around others like themselves, perhaps work among whites, and then retreat to segregated areas of the city. Once established, many sent for relatives who may not have had the same education and skills and a new class emerged with more opportunities and better employment.

The community the new Negro left behind became the home of those with no, little, or low income, education, and employment. And following the same pattern as whites, blacks with more money and education distanced themselves once more from the others, moving farther and farther away from the inner city. However, this time they did not bring their less fortunate family members into their new world of cleaner and safer schools, stores, and homes. They even formed their own neighborhoods just for those who had moved up the financial ladder. Seeking to assimilate to the white lifestyle, they did not realize or perhaps care about the effect that distancing themselves would create. Even today, there is still a continuous motion as whites move out of neighborhoods when blacks move in. And then middle- to upper-class blacks move out when other blacks, whom they view as lesser than them and a threat to their status, move in.

Left behind in the inner cities were largely people who had arrived unprepared and under-skilled. Some well-intended social programs were tried, but failed from a lack of understanding, an inability to establish effective communication and interaction, and little if any follow-through. Initially planned as temporary, huge housing projects became virtual holding cells that imprisoned people physically, mentally, and emotionally. Poor schools, lack of resources, high unemployment, lower incomes, and other realities contributed to the decline in inner cities that continues today. Communities once bustled with family-owned businesses and factory jobs. Now those are gone. Corner grocery stores now sell liquor. Barbershops, if they are even open, have too many empty chairs. The tailors and dry cleaners have left and there are few pharmacies. Factory jobs, while often low-paying, did offer a living wage. Now empty, towering structures are homes for vagrants and drug users instead of workers sewing, assembling, packing, or processing.

Inner cities grew poorer as business and employment moved too far away for inner-city residents to reach without public transportation or cars. With the loss of these opportunities, people also lost their work ethic, skills, and self-esteem. Many believe that some companies do not list entry-level jobs in the newspaper, especially the black community newspapers, as a way to screen out inner-city residents, who increasingly perceive that they have been written off as unemployable. Unfortunately, they begin to believe this and stop seeking employment. Without jobs, the residents obviously cannot support local businesses, and the stores that remain offer the cheapest, lowest-quality products available. Many merchants simply do not care if what they sell is outdated, spoiled, or damaged.

So, inner cities have many people with insecurities and a lack of trust, high unemployment, low-education levels, few and poor resources, premature death rates, and unnecessary health problems. Yet these are the people who are supposed to move us through the next century and produce offspring to help lead the country. In the past, black families have faced numerous situations that threatened their survival, but that was before the onslaught of crime, drugs, disease, and a lack of concern about life that have already wiped out thousands of people and threaten to do more harm if not stopped. It seems as if inner-city residents are the least cared-about people in the United States. In fact, I think some people do not even see them or consider their importance to this country. Of what we see and hear about—the one or two homeless people begging for money on the street, youths killed every weekend, drug addicts overdosing, and those who die young of illnesses and leave unhealthy children behind to become wards of the state—there are hundreds of thousands more who are invisible to us. Tall buildings, bridges, subway tracks, concrete walls and other barriers have surrounded them and hide them.

In 1999, the U.S. Census Bureau reported that 55 percent of African

Americans lived in cities, compared to only 22 percent of whites. According to *The African American Internetwork,* (www.afamnet.com, March 7, 2000) the top 10 metropolitan areas where African Americans lived in 1996 were, in order of their populations, New York, Chicago, Detroit, Philadelphia, Los Angeles, Houston, Baltimore, the District of Columbia, Memphis, and New Orleans. How will these residents help you when you are a senior citizen? Will they be trained as nurses or dieticians? Will they be able to correct the problems in their own communities? Considering the high rates of murder, suicide, and premature deaths from poor health or lack of treatment, will they even be here? Think about these questions from a view other than race, culture, and class. These questions are about the survival of the United States.

Inner-City Blues

For some it is easier to emphasize and focus on the positive, but there is no way to help the inner city without dealing directly with the true scope of the crisis. Yes, what is presented here may have been mentioned before, but when looking at the magnitude of the problems one shudders. Further, what is described below is just a short list of what plagues the inner cities.

We can characterize the quality of life for most of America's inner-city residents as darker than blue, more black and bleak. The sadness is that many of these people are like the 12 lost tribes of Israel, who wandered aimlessly for 40 years because they had lost their faith and hope. Likewise, many inner-city dwellers in the United States are lost. They do not have a vision of hope and of what is possible. They see and experience a series of failures and obstacles, reinforced by society. African Americans have survived the horrific conditions of slavery, forced segregation, and then economic dependence on a society that is ready to pull the rug out from under them. The family structure has been broken altogether because African American men are not present and both men and women are not following God's standards for relationships and other behaviors and responsibilities. Their creativity, resourcefulness, productivity, independence, and labor have been stripped away, leaving them with no self-esteem or motivation. They do not see models of integrity, morality, commitment, and service. The role models that were historically part of the black community have moved away. A typical inner-city household is overcrowded with several families or generations living together. Ten children and four adults may reside in a three-bedroom apartment. The adults may be drug users and unemployed and are probably high school dropouts. Any older children will have also already dropped out and started using drugs. An unmarried female teenager may have one or two children. Nutrition and hygiene are poor. The house is not kept clean and someone is always sick. The lack of privacy means that there is no space for children to study even if they tried. There may be a television and stereo, but no basic educational tools such as pencils, paper, or books. The children are perhaps a grade or two behind academically and behind others their same age developmentally. This group of 10 has moved at least three times in the past year and there is frequent arguing because no one has a space of his or her own. There is never enough of anything, including food and money.

Why are we concerned? Why should you be concerned? The answer to both questions is elementary. Economic and physical distress cuts across all races and cultural lines. However, it does seem to have boundaries that envelop the inner city, primarily because of the high concentration of the most vulnerable people. Despite their location, status, or cultural identity, they are people just like we are and deserve better options, treatment, care, and attention. Whether we like it or not, the residents in these areas often seen by others as less than desirable, make up a large portion of this country's population. With its high birth rates and steady influx of new residents, especially immigrants, the inner city will ultimately comprise the largest segment of America's population. We have seen the serious results of widespread poverty in Third-World countries. Now, the United States has similar conditions in its own cities. Without strong, healthy people living in suitable conditions, how can we grow as a nation or even keep up or compete with others? We cannot. All of us have something to give, offer, or suggest, but more important we have an obligation to help others. Through the partnering described in this book, one can begin to see how much we can accomplish when we work together. We need to break the oppressive chains of the destitute, disenfranchised, and underserved people. We have to unlock their minds, nurture them, and give them wisdom if we are relying on them to carry this country forward through the 21st century. There are many chains, some self-imposed and others not, with too many locks. Yet we hold the keys. As long as they are virtual hostages, unhealthy conditions will persist. It is said that "the truth shall set you free." Full recognition of how the problems of others affect you today and tomorrow will free you to do what is necessary to release and help others.

The Boiling Pot

The change from an industrial economy to one that is high-tech has affected the inner-city neighborhoods where manufacturing was one of the primary sources for employment. In many of those once bustling communities, unemployment rates are higher than the national average and residents do not share in the country's recent prosperity. The U.S. Department of Labor's 1999 *Report on the American Workforce* revealed that the gaps in wages between more- and less-educated workers remain large and that much of the growth has been in temporary and part-time positions, which carry low wages and benefits and are insufficient to provide even the basics for a family. These jobs offer the poor no hope for long-term, livable employment. Also overlooked are those out-of-work Americans who have simply given up on finding jobs.

The health status of urban communities falls below that of the rest of the population. Home to 30 percent of all Americans, according to 1999 U.S. Census Bureau estimates, large, urban areas are breeding grounds for the most deadly germs known and some not yet identified. While big cities may have the best hospitals with the brightest doctors, crowding makes it easy for germs to spread through direct or indirect contact. As cities have grown, bacteria, viruses, parasites, and contagious illnesses have become resistant to drugs, and social conditions have contributed to the rise and prevalence of noncommunicable diseases such as heart disease as well.

Many studies have shown that minority and low-income communities are more likely to be exposed to serious environmental hazards and health risks. The Commission for Racial Justice of the United Church of Christ released a report in 1987 (and updated in 1994), *Toxic Wastes and Race in the United States,* which found that the areas with the most commercial hazardous-waste sites had higher proportions of racial minorities. These medically underserved populations also have less access to information and political influence to help them oppose and correct these injustices.

Young African Americans perhaps face the greatest threats to their health. Although overall infant mortality rates in the United States have declined in the last 30 years, the National Center for Health Statistics reported that in 1997 black infants continued to die at twice the rate of white infants. Death caused by disorders related to low birth weight, one of the leading causes of infant mortality, was four times more likely among African Americans. Similarly, while the average blood lead levels in the United States declined through the 1990s, exposure to lead remained a major environmental disease for African American children. The U.S. Department of Housing and Urban Development's 1997 report *Moving Toward a Lead-Safe America* reported that 22 percent of young African Americans living in large central cities had blood lead levels exceeding the level of concern set by the Centers for Disease Control and Prevention (CDC). Left untreated, high levels of lead exposure can affect a child's nervous system resulting in aggressiveness, inability to concentrate, and a reduced intelligence level. Severe cases can result in seizures, comas, and kidney disease.

Violent crime among teenagers, both perpetrators and victims, continues to be of urgent concern, particularly in the African American community. Data from the CDC's National Center for Injury Prevention and Control showed that in 1997 homicide was the leading cause of death for African American males between the ages of 15 and 24. The overwhelming majority of these young men were killed with firearms. Suicide among the young has also been on the rise. The Surgeon General's *Call to Action to Prevent Suicide, 1999,* listed suicide as the third leading cause of death for Americans between the ages of 15 and 24. From 1980–1996 the highest increase in suicide rates—105 percent—has been among young African American males. These deaths stem from a combination of sociological, psychological, and biological factors. Among youth, alcohol abuse, drug dependency, depression, and behavioral problems contribute to the high rate of suicide cited by the Surgeon General.

The National Institute on Alcohol Abuse and Alcoholism reported at the end of 1999 that approximately one in four children in the United States is exposed at some time before the age of 18 to family alcohol abuse or alcoholism. The findings, published in the *American Journal of Public Health* (Vol. 90, No. 1), underscore the enormous impact this has on the nation's youth, making children vulnerable to medical, cognitive, emotional, and behavioral problems. Marital conflict compounds the problem. School records show children of alcoholics have greater academic difficulties, such as repeating grades and dropping out of school, and more referrals to school psychologists. These children often exhibit behaviors that include lying, stealing, fighting, and general conduct problems.

The National Center for Health Statistics released data in 1999 revealing higher rates of out-of-wedlock birth among African American women: 69 percent in 1997, compared to the national rate of 32 percent. Many of these women and their children are among the unacceptably high number of Americans who are homeless. In 1999 the Department of Housing and Urban Development released a comprehensive report, *The Forgotten Americans—Homelessness: Programs and the People They Serve.* Among its findings were that 71 percent of homeless people live in central cities and 40 percent of the homeless population is made up of families with children. These children have been through the unimaginable, including domestic abuse and sleeping on relatives' floors, before ending up totally homeless. They suffer physically, cognitively, and emotionally.

Other studies have shown that black children are more at risk for mental retardation and other developmental disabilities, often partly because of the conditions mentioned above. The Metropolitan Atlanta Developmental Disabilities Study, a long-term, collaborative project by the federal government, state agencies, and Emory University, has studied the prevalence of these diseases in school-aged children. The results thus far have indicated that rates of mental retardation are higher among African American children, and that mothers with low education levels were more likely to have a child with mental retardation.

We frequently read about the poor dietary habits of American children, and in this area African American children often fare worse than their white counterparts. In just one example, an article in the journal *Preventive Medicine* (1990 July; 19(4): 432-42) showed how differences in dietary patterns between the races also has implications for disease prevention. Among children ages 1 to 17, black children had higher cholesterol and fat intakes, which are much less favorable for cardiovascular health.

Children are not the only members of the African American community whose health is at risk. Lack of proper health care and health maintenance among seniors and the homeless in inner cities results in unnecessary deaths. For older citizens, the Centers for Disease Control recommends flu vaccines as the most important preventive measure to protect individuals from the serious complications of the influenza virus, including death from pneumonia. Crowded living conditions among high-risk populations help viruses spread rapidly.

Certain ailments that frequently lead to serious complications are known to be more prevalent among African Americans. According to the National Eye Institute, glaucoma is the leading cause of blindness among African Americans, who are three to four times more likely to develop glaucoma and six times more likely to become blind from the disease than whites. Many people at higher risk are unaware of the importance of early detection—through regular eye examinations—and an estimated one in eight African Americans will have the disease by the age of 70. And the 1998 American Lung Association Asthma Survey confirmed the findings of other studies that the impact of the disease is much greater on African American families than among whites. In the mid-1990s, asthma rates were over 20 percent higher among African Americans and they accounted for a similar percentage of asthma-related deaths. These deaths are preventable with a simple asthma management plan, which should include limiting and eliminating attack triggers such as rodent urine, cockroaches, animal dander, dust mites, and secondhand smoke.

The National Prostate Cancer Coalition reported in early 2000 that African American men have the highest prostate cancer incidence and mortality rates in the world. In 1999, it was the most commonly detected cancer and the second-leading cause of cancer deaths among African American males. Unfortunately, most men do not know they have the disease because they do not get regular prostate exams and the cancer grows without noticeable symptoms or problems for months to years. Diabetes also places a heavy toll on the African American community. The African American Program of the American Diabetes Association provides information and education on the impact of this disease, which affects an estimated 10 percent of all African Americans and 25 percent between the ages of 65 and 74. African Americans are 1.7 times more likely to have either Type I or Type II diabetes than whites and experience higher rates of the serious complications of the disease: blindness, amputations, heart attack, and end-stage renal disease. African American women are most at risk as are those who have a family history of the disease.

Obesity is a contributing risk factor to diabetes, and to other diseases such as hypertension and heart disease. It is a growing problem throughout the entire U.S. population and especially among male and female residents of inner-city environments, ultimately taking a toll on the health of the community. Factors commonly associated with an increase in the prevalence of obesity include poverty, low education levels, inactivity, and genetics. Higher obesity rates are more common among women in minority ethnic groups. According to the National Center for Health Statistics, although the average national rate among adults was 33 percent between 1988 and 1991, the rate among African American women was almost 50 percent.

On average, the life expectancy of African Americans is currently six-plus years less than that of whites, according to the December 13, 1999, *National Vital Statistics Report* (Vol. 47, No. 28) from the National Center for Health Statistics. African American males have a life expectancy of 67.2 compared to 74.3 for white men and African American women have a life expectancy of 74.7 compared to 79.7 for white women.

Consider what it is like to live in a community with just half of this short list of health, environmental, and social problems. Would you be able to thrive? Would you be healthy, hopeful, and happy? I do not think so. In reviewing a few of the issues and problems facing residents of inner cities, it is clear they are deeply rooted in social, economic, and political realities that churches, universities, human-service agencies, and other institutions can help eradicate. One may ask, where has the church been all of this time? Why has the church let these conditions occur and continue? What all parties have to realize is that the same economic, social, education, and environmental conditions affect the church. If a plant closes, church giving goes down, members move to another area, and corporate support decreases. Meanwhile, the community's needs increase and the church has to provide more and different services. If the neighborhood has high crime and drug abuse levels, then the church and its members have been affected or victimized, but the church itself has not moved, it is where it has always been and still strives to serve the community.

What is important to remember is that African Americans want the healing powers found in the comfort of churches, and seek out church leaders for practically every situation or problem that arises. There is growing interest among medical and public health researchers in the powerful connections between health and spirituality and religious participation, areas that have often been overlooked by the medical establishment in the past. Some recent studies have examined the link between participation in religious services and health status and the role that prayer, church attendance, and a relationship with God can play in the reduction of high blood pressure and other serious diseases. Many involved in this field believe that faith and prayer can play an important role in avoiding, reducing, or eliminating drug and alcohol abuse, suicide, and juvenile delinquency, and prayer or meditation can help patients relax, decrease heart and breathing rates, and reduce muscle tension. This connection has been helpful in cases of both non-life-threatening and serious illnesses, such as cancer and AIDS.

Spirituality, faith, prayer and religion have proven to have a healing and healthy impact on people's lives. Best of all, there are no negative side effects and it is safe, free, and available to everyone. The combination of the church's firm standing and its history of taking care of the community—and, of course, its spiritual benefits—make it an important conduit to people who are typically hard to reach by outsiders. However, churches cannot address all of the needs alone and neither can any other group. Churches need resources to back up their presence, history, track record, and ability to influence change. Churches want to play a proactive role in dealing with the economic depression, the environmental land mines, the health crisis, the drug epidemic, the crime battlefield, and more. Just having service on Sunday is not enough, nor is it the desire of the churches and congregations. The ministers and congregations of the churches see the devastating results of the problems every day, with condemned buildings falling down around them, youth without jobs or a safe place to go, drug and alcohol use, poor health conditions, trash along the streets, homelessness, and entirely too many funerals for young people. A lot of these things have been said before at one time or another, but is anyone really listening? Is anyone ready to work toward ending widespread health and social conditions that ultimately affect all of us? It is time to make a long-term commitment to change this "community-of-emergency" wherever it may be and among whatever race. We must erase the term "urban underclass" from our minds, vocabulary, sight, and our future.

Collectively, churches have a powerful network, a vocal press, political influence, national and community-based affiliations and organizations, voting power, cultural knowledge, and, most important, community trust. Even with these strengths, the massiveness of the issues and the different populations affected dictates that efforts to bring about change have to be equally massive. Further, they have to be accepted by the leaders of different populations, whether Asian, Haitian, American Indian, Hispanic, or African American. This is not simple rhetoric. By enlarging the scope, the tools and skills for positive change are within our hands. Change is attainable wherever people are willing to see these challenges as opportunities. This book describes what is critical to addressing these challenges and proposes pursuing a strategic, bottom-line, results-oriented relationship between the church, community, hospitals, and other institutions. With this alignment, problems that seem as large as Goliath can be knocked out by a group of Davids.

CHAPTER TWO

Churches Collaborating for Change

As DISCUSSED IN CHAPTER ONE, inner cities face numerous challenges. Yet these challenges can be overcome through collaborative
relationships and projects, especially those involving the church.
Speaking directly to church leaders now, most of you know firsthand
that decreasing government funding for human services combined
with increasing social problems have turned our inner cities into dis-
mal dungeons of despair for those who live there as well as those
who live and work around these areas. Nowhere are preventable,
treatable, and controllable health and social problems so rampant. As
church leaders, you have always exercised your God-driven directive
to supply not just the spiritual needs of the congregation and community, but all of the other "people" needs as well. However, those
"people" needs keep increasing while your resources continue to
decrease. Now, if your community is like most inner-city communities it is in crisis, losing a battle for survival. This is a crisis that the
church cannot fight alone. The changing nature of America's inner
cities and the shifting nature of life and death health issues, without
even considering crime, dictate a new response. As pastors and active
church leaders, you have seen the social fabric of our country torn.
The social fabric of the inner cities is already in shreds. The family
unit is rarely seen and families that can only be characterized as sur-
vivors are banding together. Immigrants and minority ethnic groups
add to the diversity of our communities, but also add different needs
and interests. The church is challenged to allocate dwindling resources
to growing problems. To be effective and survive you must go
beyond the congregation, offering the basic social services and reach

out to people and organizations that can help the church bring positive change to the whole community.

While the church has been self-sufficient in many ways and not one to ask for help, it is time to fulfill its mission by going beyond the doors of the church and up to the doors of the ivory towers and knocking real hard. A common saying is, "all they can do is to say no," or "you will never know if you don't ask." But don't view asking as begging for a handout. What you are looking for is a handshake, or a high five, symbolizing an agreement to work together to address problems in your community. Not taking this important and for many unprecedented step diminishes the ability of the church to do its job, resulting in further problems inside and beyond the church walls. What harms the community harms the church; what benefits the community benefits the church. This should encourage you to form alliances that can affect the future of both the community and the church. View the alliance as planting a seed and then nurturing it to grow and be fruitful. Remember that everyone who shares a concern or benefits from the community in some way should bear the responsibility for the social conditions within that community. In this case, "everyone" includes hospitals, public and private agencies, the government, and civic and business leaders. The burden can no longer rest only with the churches.

These types of alliances have gained momentum in recent years, as churches, community groups, and institutions that serve the same people search for more effective ways to promote public health and enhance the quality of life in the community. Further, an alliance with an institution or any other organization allows both partners to improve and expand the quality of services provided. While the collaborative approach is still evolving, a basic understanding of how to work together, which issues to address, and organizational considerations are common to all collaborations. Critical to the collaboration is recognition that the relationship has to be fostered and that it is a learning process for all participants. While both sides have specific responsibilities and strengths, all will share in the successes, failures, and frustrations that will occur throughout the relationship. Without this, the relationship will not develop to maturity. The goal is to view each other not as sides, but as partners.

While there are advantages to forming an alliance, there are some disadvantages as well. You need to weigh these and decide if a collaboration is right for you and the members of the church. Are you willing to share the responsibility, the accountability, the recognition, and the possible negative reaction? Is the church in agreement and totally supportive of partnering? Some advantages are that the combined resources allow activities to take place that a single organization could not undertake; both partners can benefit from each other's strengths; alliances generally get more respect and are taken seriously; and collaborations can overcome roadblocks to gain access that leads to accomplishments. On the other hand, when you work with another group you simply cannot make decisions as you are accustomed. You may find the coalition time consuming and labor-intensive. You will have to compromise and lead your congregation or other volunteers to do the same. Also, with any group of people there will be different levels of commitment, consistency, resources, skills, and, of course, personalities. What is required here is a reality and an ego check!

Before the seed can grow, you must undertake a lot of groundwork as you will probably be dealing with soil that has never been tilled before. Planning and cultivation are essential to the success of the alliance's harvest. Begin the planning process with research. Take a look around the community and determine what issues the church would like to address; there are many and you have to narrow your focus at first. You may decide to deal with diabetes, lead poisoning, or nutrition issues. Or you may be contacted by an institution that has already identified an area in which it wants to work. You will then have to decide if its focus is one in which you, your congregation, and supporters can assist effectively and whether the focus will negatively impact the beliefs or practices of the church. For example, the project may relate to abortion or birth control in a manner that is opposite the beliefs of the church. Certainly, you will be clear in your doctrine, but if there is any hesitation get input from the congregation and other ministry leaders. Without their support, neither the collaboration nor the project will work.

For relationships you initiate yourself, you must first have a clear picture of what you want to address, how you can assist another group or institution, and how their involvement can assist your church and community. Then you need to identify what institution(s) can realistically help the community through the church. Think about ways to bring the plight of your community to their attention and keep the communication flowing. Become a resource of information and offer to help, even if it is not for the project you have in mind. Institutions looking for partners, particularly those in the health and human service areas, are seeking community-based organizations to work closely with them to improve the functional status and results of community public health activities. Two fairly common goals are reorienting public health programs and services toward community needs and concerns, and ensuring that community-based organizations play a key role in shaping public health services and working with health professionals. The institutions are interested in an established organization or a respected community leader with a track record of making things happen both within and outside of the community. They also want the community to take an active role in assessing its own needs as a way of guaranteeing that local priorities are addressed, while giving special attention to specific needs. The structure should stress teamwork among public health educators, professionals, and community leaders. Additionally, ongoing education and leadership training for public health employees and community volunteers is a goal shared by both partners.

Churches are somewhat behind in tapping into the existing and future resources available through collaborating with other institutions and organizations. Whether or not a given project comes to fruition, ultimately these institutions will help you when the right project and funding come along. Many organizations have longtime partners that have coauthored grant requests and, in general, know the approach and what is desired in a partner. These are things that church leaders and administrators need to learn quickly. In most cases, because of such collaborations more support will become available from foundations and public grants sooner than you think.

So, how do you begin? Believe it or not, you start by looking at yourself and the church body. Is this really something you want to do? If so, you may need to position the church as one that is available, proactive, and receptive to collaborations. It will be important to reinforce or build the reputation of the church and church leadership. Take advantage of opportunities for visibility among those with whom you would like to partner, those who have relationships with potential partners, and, most of all, the community. You want organizations and people to know that you are open to adding or assisting with new services and that you can meet their needs. Further, you want to differentiate your church and yourself from others. You must have established your credibility and deliverability before you approach an institution or before one would seriously consider partnering with your church. You do realize that the institution will look at you through one of the most powerful microscopes possible. Make sure they get a good, clear view because the community's opportunity may be riding on you! If there are things outside organizations need to know about, tell them first before they hear about it elsewhere.

At the same time that you are looking at yourself, start looking closely at possible partners. Consider health and health-related organizations, philanthropic organizations, educational institutions, public health professional associations, and community-based organizations, among the range of possibilities. Then ask questions and investigate. What is their reputation in the community? Have they done community work before? Do they have allies or enemies in the community? If feasible, look at another community in which they did work to determine what was expected and what was the outcome. Would that community accept them back?

The first direct questions should include: Why do you want to do this project? What is your organization going to gain by doing this project? What are you going to gain personally? How is the community going to benefit during and after the project? What is your level of commitment to this project and community? Is this the first of other potential projects or a one-time only project? Why did you choose me and my church? How do you expect us to help? What is your idea of a partnership? Of course, there are lots of other questions that will lead to yet more questions. Once again, if you don't ask you will never know. And, in this case, not knowing can be disastrous. In the previous chapter, I referred to the relationship like a marriage. Well, now I would say the beginning of the relationship is like a father questioning his only daughter's husband-to-be, whom he has never met or even heard of before. There is nothing wrong with being cautious and protective. African Americans in particular have been too often misled, tricked, used, and, as we sometimes say, have gotten the short end of the stick; because someone did not double check what was being said or promised, there were no checks and balances put in place. The result is a lack of trust in any group coming into the community to do human service-related work.

In this context, trust is a triple-sided issue. First, you have to gain the trust of the institution. Second, you have to trust the institution. Third, you have to instill trust in the institution and collaboration among your congregation and the community. From the view of the partner(s), they need assurances that you can deliver what you say you can and within the time frame needed and a demonstration of your commitment from the standpoint of time, availability, leadership, attitude toward decentralization, and reaction to problem-solving efforts. Representatives of the institution(s) will want to know if they have your full and true support. Without you personally demonstrating your trust in them, it will be difficult for the project to get off the ground. Plus, you will simply not be able to rally the support or volunteers you need to be a full-fledged partner. Putting your trust in the institution is a judgment call you have to make, and one that should not be taken lightly as you will be judged on any perceived improprieties of your partner. Further, you have to demonstrate your trust in the partner by providing them with information and access, recognizing them formally and introducing them to others, and always giving them due credit. You will want to ask your potential partner the questions listed earlier, however, in most cases you can use your God-given sense of discernment to determine whether or not to form the relationship. If you do not feel the "fit" is right, wait until you can help create another opportunity.

Partnership Development

So, you have found the right "fit" and believe that you, your church, and the institution can impact the community with a collaborative effort. Now what?

Jointly, you want to establish a partnership structure, a vision, and a mission statement with the objectives, desired outcomes, and expectations of each participating alliance member. From your standpoint, you may want the plans to include general training, training in recruiting and motivating volunteers, mentoring for youth, encouragement to enter health professions, employment and networking opportunities, cultural diversity training for those associated with the partner, and, most important, a "leave behind" component for the community.

A model community health development plan may include:

- Quality care for each person, from seniors to children.
- Ongoing care available before, during, and after an illness.
- Regularly scheduled appointments.
- Health assessments available throughout the community at various locations and convenient times.
- Health care teams for managed care, coordination, and accessibility.

- Efficient services, operations, administration, finances, and staff.
- Safe, clean sites and linkages between sites.
- Linkages with other organizations and service providers.

Until you are clear as to what the plan includes, you should not announce the partnership or plan or make promises and recruit volunteers. In establishing the structure, determine decision-making procedures, reporting requirements, and accounting processes. Think about everything that could possibly create a problem and address those things now. Be realistic in establishing the game rules and how you can play. If you know you cannot commit to personally being at every training session, then make sure that is understood and that it is okay to send a church representative. If necessary, develop a policies and procedures manual so there will be no selective memory losses. Above all, you don't want to get midway through the project and then argue over administrative issues that may impair the project and the relationship. While you have immediate outcomes you would like to see, keep in mind that your partner is looking not only to provide a medical service, but also to change existing internal and external policies. They want to refine what they do, to train and retrain community health professionals, and to come away with an expanded understanding of helping underserved populations. Remember that the service goal may be the same, but both of you have somewhat different agendas. However, these differences will ultimately help both partners and, more importantly, the community. Realizing this should help you be more accommodating, understanding, and patient with what may seem to be an endless process of recording and reporting, along with a rotation of workers that may force you to start from the very beginning at each stage. But realize the importance of what you are doing, because it may favorably impact similar communities throughout the United States. The more you can help, the more such efforts will contribute to the improvement of the delivery of health and other social services to the community, better living conditions, and lives saved.

Changing Minds in Challenging Times

Once you have formed the relationship and worked out the details, you will have to sell the collaboration and project to others. This is one of the most important things the partner expects from you as a religious leader. What is covered here can be applied to most programs prior to and during implementation.

Maybe you will be fortunate and have an easy sell. If you are less fortunate, you have to work within the congregation and encourage them to work throughout the community to build a level of acceptance of the institution. What is important here is that you, as the religious leader, have to take the lead. Not that people do not respect your assistants, but they are looking first at you for your nod of approval and your efforts to spread the word. The community, as a group of people, is probably the hardest ground to break. Some will agree almost immediately and others will require some time and interaction before they feel even remotely comfortable with the partners(s) and the project(s). The trust level will rise once the congregation and community see representatives of the institution interacting with church members and community residents.

During this time, conduct activities to share and build understanding and a common goal for the project. Introduce the community health workers to members of the community from different backgrounds—career, educational, religious, social, financial, and ethnic. Let them spend a complete day with you, so they will understand the diversity of the demands made upon you and the amount of time you spend each day ministering to the needs of the entire community. If you already have social service programs in place, such as feeding the homeless or seniors, bring the community health workers so they start gaining visibility and interacting comfortably with the resident population. Provide opportunities for the health workers to discuss concerns with the public and show they are sincere about finding ways to address problems directly or indirectly. People will not participate if they feel that their concerns are not considered important. The concerns raised and the priority of the concerns may not match what the project is intended to address. Some communities have long-established concerns centered around racial, ethnic, occupational, or neighborhood issues. Others form and reform as you solicit input. Interest groups within the community can be in opposition to each other, especially in multicultural inner cities. These multiple concerns and occasional conflicts need to be dealt with early in order to develop a skillful, sensitive strategy to introduce the program effectively. Both partners must help build cooperative bonds needed for lasting relationships that encompass all elements of the community and center around its fundamental concerns. It may be necessary to consider widening the scope of the project or bringing in other resources for hands-on assistance or referrals. The broadened outlook recognizes the value of activities and conditions that contribute to the acceptance and eventual implementation of the project. In summary, community-exposure actions help the community health workers become accustomed to the community's lifestyles, concerns, interests, and cultures. With your help, the community health workers get to feel the pulse of the community, while finding out what makes the community tick.

This process is key for the development of introductory materials to recruit community health workers, volunteers, and individuals to serve on an advisory board or board of directors for the project(s). The materials should be brief and to the point. The two issues that need to be addressed first are "What are we (the church and community) getting out of this project?" and "What are you getting out of this project?" As someone who already interacts with the community, you can advise partners on how to phrase their responses appropriately and what types of information to disseminate, what questions are likely to be asked, and the best format to use for sharing the information. You may decide that one-on-one meetings with leave-behind material, combined with presentations to community organizations and clubs, are the most effective way to get the word out. Or, you may suggest sending information to all churches in the community for inclusion in church bulletins and posting on bulletin boards. A series of open, community-wide meetings may be what your particular community is accustomed to for obtaining information. Regardless of the chosen method of communication, the method and materials have to be tailored to the audience. While the institution may want to produce a slick direct mail piece or poster, if you know these are not effective advise them to stick with what people are accustomed to seeing. Just because what the community uses now is not slick does not mean it is not effective and that point needs to be made. The community also wants an effective approach.

Additionally, you and members of your congregation or ministry team need to review all materials before distribution. I would go as far as to suggest even reviewing speeches prior to speaking engagements. One slip of the tongue, use of the wrong word, or condescending joke could cause problems even before the project begins. For example, you know that most African Americans are offended if someone of another race says "you people." Those simple words are fighting words and will create unrest. You know the buzz words that the audience will or will not understand and that it is not interested in receiving information riddled with the slang that most find useless, offensive, and wish would disappear. Trying to be hip is not the way. Although the institution's staff must know what terms or slang mean, this doesn't mean that they should try to use something that is not natural to them personally or the institution they represent. The institution must rely on you for help in this area and you must insist on prior approval. The materials developed must complement and build upon recruitment efforts.

To insure a smooth transition from project concept to implementation, consider creating a broad-based task force that could be divided into a number of committees, including accounting, community relations, media relations, policies and procedures, health administration, and reporting to funding sources. If you do this, it is essential to include representatives from the community. While a chairperson could track and coordinate each committee's activities, there should be no rank within the committees; they should be seen as equal resources for advice and consultation. You don't want to establish another class or authoritative level. All participants should understand and share the ultimate goals of the project.

Recruiting Volunteers

Again, this is an area in which the institution will rely heavily on your help. Only you and your church leaders know whom to approach in the congregation and community. The institution trusts you to recommend good candidates, so you must first screen potential candidates. Issues to consider include whether the person has volunteered before in the church or community; is respected in the church and among the community; has applicable skills and will accept direction; is willing to attend training sessions and can commit the necessary amount of time; and has worked with a group before and is capable of obtaining the information and communicating it with others. The last thing you want is a person who feels slighted and will negatively influence others' participation and cooperation.

Recruiting of volunteers should begin in your own church. Obviously, you know the members and they know you, and if they agree to participate they won't let you down. Their involvement gives the church a greater sense of ownership and pride in the project. If you have to go beyond the congregation, ask members for suggestions; they will recommend people whom they trust and believe will not embarrass them by failing to follow through. Recruiting can be formal with kick-off events or less formal by messages from the pulpit, sign-up sheets, announcements in the church bulletin, and letters and telephone calls. When recruiting in front of an audience, if possible have representatives of the institution or the assigned community health worker(s) present, so people will begin to associate names with faces. Many times people are reluctant to sign up for anything until they can ask some questions. You might want them to indicate an interest and then meet with all those interested as a group or individually to secure their involvement. Issues that should be addressed include time availability, scheduling, organizational support, the availability of backup, the working conditions, the kind of work entailed, the ability to make decisions or deviate from the directives, the commitment required, safety issues, and the possible psychological effects. Once again, have representatives of the institution involved in this process as much as possible; however, if you think their presence will inhibit the open exchange of questions, you might opt not to have them present at first.

After selecting volunteers, it is time for training. You will need a curriculum for a training session, including all copies of forms and questions for the volunteers. Like all written materials, this must be reviewed by you and others within your church for cultural sensitivity, linguistics, and acceptable processes. You should request that the training take place at the church or another convenient, non-threatening place. You or a representative of the church should lead the session, with back-up assistance from the community health workers and health providers. The initial training should be directed at managers and supervisors to prepare them to relay information and respond properly to those they supervise. They must become skilled in team building, motivation, administration, problem solving, mentoring, and overseeing training and education. They must also meet or communicate frequently with the appropriate partnership leaders to provide feedback and updates and obtain direction and guidance. Where necessary, they need to consider suggestions regarding the expansion or revision of strategies to carry out the project. Their training should emphasize the need for them to coach, counsel, coordinate, evaluate, and troubleshoot. They should be encouraged to take initiative and depart from traditional thinking, as you are not approaching the community's problems in a traditional manner. Mistakes might be made, but this is also a sign of an honest attempt to respond to or solve a problem.

While pretesting is mandatory before starting any community project, timing is an important factor in the implementation of the plan. Implementation that moves too slowly may dampen enthusiasm and reduce momentum. Implementation that moves too quickly can create confusion and may threaten the success of the project through the use of rushed, untested, or faulty methods. With a group of volunteers, it is advisable to begin with the easier tasks to obtain some accomplishments early to keep the interest level high. This also gives you the opportunity to continue training and evaluating the volunteers. Meeting some of the easier goals may help the volunteers and partnership prepare for more complex tasks. During this start-up period, a comprehensive evaluation of the partnership is beneficial. The partners should evaluate each other; the managers and supervisors should evaluate the partners; and the volunteers should evaluate the work, communication, and training. The partners or managers and supervisors should also evaluate the volunteers, the assignments, questionnaires, data recording methods, and other organizational matters. A comprehensive analysis across all areas is essential to guide the effort to its most effective and efficient level of operation.

In addition to assessing the project's impact on the community, you should also look for positive changes among the group. Among those you can expect to see are an increased level of participation and cooperation; contacts between volunteers, community health workers, and health providers; application of training and an increased sense of the importance of the work; a greater belief in citizen involvement in problem solving; a sense of partnering and relationships among the volunteers; and suggestions for action beyond what has been asked. Now, all these things may not happen or may not happen at once. However, if there is any discontent, deal with the problem or person immediately. Certainly not everyone will be buddies, but as the saying goes, don't let one bad apple spoil the whole bunch. You may also find that some people may be getting burned out or too involved personally in the participants' lives and situations. You may have to pull that volunteer out of the program totally or temporarily. For this reason, it is advisable to have trained backup available so the work can continue.

Checks and Balances

Any project and partnership must have checks and balances in the form of evaluations, reports, tracking methods, and other means to routinely monitor all aspects of the relationship and goals. Relevant evaluation measures include how well the volunteers have bonded with other volunteers, how they have formed relationships with community residents, and their understanding of the importance of their contributions to the team. Since it is a team effort, evaluate the team in terms of its functioning. Some changes may be needed as trends are revealed. For instance, a volunteer may go to a home to collect data that should require at best 15 minutes to obtain. However, upon entering the home, she finds a single, elderly person who has an immediate need that has to be met, such as ordering medicine from a pharmacy, cleaning up a spill, or taking out the trash. Fifteen minutes can be spent just being respectful and looking at pictures of grandchildren. While these actions may keep the volunteer from seeing as many people as planned that day, it will guarantee an open door for a return visit and a positive word about the project to other community residents.

Methods for evaluating the partnership overall should reflect the goals and objectives for the project. Check to see if the project is on schedule and if the church and partner have done what they agreed to do from the onset. If necessary and appropriate make or request changes in the schedule. But try not to view the need to make such changes as a failure. Sometimes this is the only way you can truly succeed at what you are trying to accomplish.

CHAPTER THREE

Interaction and Communication with Churches and Inner-City Communities

For any organization desiring to work with churches, effective interaction involves learning about the church and the community challenges, partnering with the right church for the needs of the project, understanding how best to implement the project and reach the community without offense, and skillful marketing. Books could be written on each of these areas; however, this chapter provides a basic start toward forging an effective relationship with all participants—from the project staff to the recipients of care.

Additionally, effective interaction with inner-city populations depends upon understanding that models, strategies, or techniques that have been successful in rural, suburban, or middle- to upper-class communities are not effective when implemented in inner cities. Each environment presents its own unique challenges. Accordingly, community health workers must fully recognize and address the special challenges faced when working within inner cities. Appropriate actions are critical to success in working within these important communities, home to millions of our nation's population.

The first and perhaps biggest challenge, though, is self-reflection to confront misconceptions, biases, and misinformation that may inhibit reaching established goals. A sincere commitment must be made to changing the way things are viewed. Key to this is understanding cultural differences between white and African Americans, acknowledging the hesitancy of African Americans to trust whites, accepting everyone as equal but perhaps as having different experiences or purposes, and, above all, working through the communication channels that are unique to African American inner-city communities.

Having considered all there is to learn, one may think that interacting with African Americans effectively is nearly impossible or difficult, particularly in inner cities. Untrue! First, plug in by learning how the community operates. This takes groundwork, beginning on sacred ground: the churches within the community.

The churches are key sources of educators, communicators, mobilizers, and others with influence in the African American community, even among non-church members. Ministers, preachers, pastors, bishops, and other religious leaders interact with the entire community, not only with those who enter the four walls of the church. They are "on call" 24 hours a day and 7 days a week. Their churches are the centers of activity and information in the communities in which they are located. In most inner cities, there is practically one church on every street. Approximately 60 percent of all Americans report belonging to a religious congregation. Among inner-city residents, about 68 percent attend church, while others visit for support services such as food banks, soup kitchens, seniors programs, or day care services. The church is the primary and in many cases the only institution that still exists in many communities. It has traditionally been a major source, sometimes the only source, of comfort and security for African Americans. Today, it remains strong and continues to grow.

From a biblical standpoint, there is a God-prescribed responsibility for religious leaders to include health and social issues in their work. In the past, many focused their efforts on overseas missions to build and operate hospitals. Now, churches and their leaders want to do the same in their own communities and they are becoming the keys to opening doors for success in inner-city health promotion and prevention programs, whether national, state, or local. Collaborating with churches to form partnerships and networks is the way to move closer to heal and save hard-to-reach, high-risk populations. Both parties have the same interests and need each other for maximum success, but collaborating can be a challenge in itself if both parties do not handle it properly.

Collaborating With the Right Church

The potential success of the program is greater with the direct involvement of the pastor. Having the involvement of the pastor or minister, rather than an associate, is critical. Generally, the associate does not have the same influence and following. A further consideration is how bureaucratic the church may be, for example, how many boards and committees are involved in making a decision. Ask how long it takes to make a decision and what steps are involved. Find out how close the pastor is to the community and how the community feels about the pastor and church. Is the church or pastor viewed as aloof or as acting superior to others? Can they really relate at the grass-roots level with the community? After talking with the pastor, don't settle for starting the program with someone from the church who may not have the contact or initial impact needed to launch a successful program. After program implementation, an associate can take over, but even then, make sure the associate is prepared, has been involved, has the same level of commitment, and is respected within and outside of the church.

In identifying the right church, talk to the pastors to find out if they really want to participate; if they can participate at the level needed; if they believe in the purpose of and goals for the project; and the extent of their commitment. A frequent mistake made by community health researchers is pursuing the largest church with the most members and a highly visible pastor. Associating with these types of churches does not automatically mean success. While many "megachurches" have strong interests in community health, they lack time to commit to the project. Additionally, some churches or church leaders will focus on forming a partnership simply to add resources to their own mission. Therefore, the partner must investigate the church just as vigorously as the church must scrutinize the organization.

The leader of a smaller congregation can probably commit to a long-term project. And ideal congregations are often the smaller, lower-income churches. Many members may receive social security, social services, disability, or have low-paying jobs. While these churches are "small" in respect to members, income, or the size of their buildings, they are "big" on actively helping each other and the surrounding community. In fact, some of the congregation may be able to participate in the research. These churches are more grass-roots and hands-on, as the congregation plays a role in maintaining the church's spiritual purpose and its physical presence. They do not have hundreds of people to rely upon to get things done, so they are action-oriented and responsible.

Find out about alliances, organized communications, or joint meetings within the community. Schedule a time to speak or to distribute information and ask interested persons to make contact directly to discuss a possible collaboration in detail. Use initial meetings to discuss the program, but more importantly to share information in a face-to-face conversation. Do not begin what might be a long-term relationship on an impersonal level.

The best test is personal contact through meetings, interviews, observation, and socializing. When talking and exploring, consider asking some of the questions below. Asking the right questions helps to bring together the best match, based upon mutual goals. The questions should include the following:

1. **How long have you been involved with this church?**
   (This will help you assess the minister's knowledge about and visibility in the community and among church membership.)

2. **Do you live in the community now, or have you lived in this community before?**
   (Church leaders with personal ties to the community may have a stronger commitment to seek change.)

3. **How many church members are active?**
   (Most important is determining how many may help with a project.)

4. What social outreach programs has the church been involved in previously?
   (Learn if the church is community-focused, open to different activities, and most important, if your project may conflict with or complement their efforts.)

5. Has the church worked with community-health professionals before?
   (This may show if the church is comfortable working with "outsiders" and sharing recognition. Find out the results of any previous partnerships and what changes, if any, would be made in hindsight.)

6. Do you have members who can help? In which areas are your members experienced (i.e., nursing, education, counseling, transportation, custodial, administration)?
   (Find out what potential resources will be available. Don't rule out any potential resources in the general congregation because they generally are the most dedicated workers, especially with training.)

7. Does your church work with other community-based or community-focused organizations?
   (Determine if the church is connected to the community outside its congregation and if it wants to work with others.)

8. Is space available for health fairs, seminars, or other activities?
   (Many members of the community, whether they attend church or not, feel more comfortable going to a church for program services and activities.)

9. What are some prominent community health problems in the neighborhood?
   (Church leaders often know more about community problems than researchers and social workers, particularly those problems that people do not report or underreport.)

10. Has the church addressed health issues previously?
    (Learn how the church has dealt with issues, the response of

the community, the obstacles, and the success. There is no need to reinvent the wheel.)

11. **How can we/I be of assistance to you, your church, and your neighborhood?**
    (In order not to be perceived as a threat or as just coming to take from the community, work toward being a true partner. Do not make false promises.)

12. **How can you be of assistance to us?**
    (Acknowledge the value of the church, its leader, and its congregation to take advantage of these untapped resources.)

13. **What other organizations or individuals do you suggest I speak with about my project?**
    (The local minister knows where the resources are within the community and will help you get a leg up on gathering information and people power.)

When questioning the church leaders, be just as prepared to answer their questions honestly and directly. To gain trust and acceptance, be straight with them and make sure the complete objectives and motives for the project are clear.

As the pastor talks, he is going to discuss both the problems of the community and those of the church. The pastor will share the needs of the church in areas such as recreation, shelter, food, housing, employment, and other social issues. To deal with the community through the church, be prepared to deal with the whole man and his problems. Be prepared to incorporate other community needs into your program; otherwise, it is not going to work.

Relationships With Clergy

Respect the minister's initial reaction and thoughts as he decides if the church will join forces with an institution. Unfortunately, from experiences that go back even further than the infamous Tuskegee

Syphilis Study, there has been a pattern of mistreatment of and dishonesty toward African Americans in heath projects. Therefore, the minister may initially be reserved and guarded. Even after an explanation of the program, there will still be some hesitancy because of the history of information being misused and capitalized upon by those other than the community assistants and research participants. The ministers know that the community health workers, researchers, and institutions gather data and publish books, and some even become famous, from information about and from African Americans and their communities. While the communities remain the same, the researcher or institution goes on to new projects. In the past, many institutions did not include service components, during or after the project. When the project ended, the institution left behind a closed door for itself and many obstacles for the next group. The minister remembers experiences like these as he considers new potential partners and projects. It is thus critical to incorporate a sustained service component to benefit the community after the project is completed. A researcher might locate a community with a high incidence of heart disease, but where will these residents go for long-term treatment when the project has ended?

The minister also thinks about how much of his own time will be required, as he already handles many roles in the church and the community. His reputation is at stake. If things do not go right, he cannot simply change positions or join a new company or profession. When the project is complete and everyone is gone, he remains and has to be able to continue his duties effectively. He needs job security just like the community health professional, especially if he joins forces with an institution with a history of community failure or mistrust.

Before and during discussions about forming a partnership, both sides must deal with the big "C" word: Control. This issue alone can doom a project before it even begins. In effect, this type of partnership is just like a marriage, requiring a level of understanding and agreement about what roles people should play, open communication, trust, honesty, equality, and achieving a mutual goal. Proper checks and balances are necessary on both ends to make sure things are going as planned. Any confusion, misunderstanding, or communication breakdown must be addressed immediately and head-on before it festers like an open wound.

Problems arise with attempts to gain control rather than work together. There cannot be hidden agendas, secret alliances, and self-serving goals; these could spell disaster for the project. Keep in mind that the pastoral partner, with his spiritual sense or intuition, knows if things are not right. And when he relays this sense to others, it sends a signal throughout the community, including other spiritual leaders and heads of organizations, and others, and the doors will close tightly. The inner-city community is open, but self-protective as well.

Community health professionals have to relinquish some control to gain the necessary acceptance, support, and information. Don't paralyze the project with the fear of losing job status by taking unfair advantage of the expertise, experience, and insight of others. Focus on the ability of the pastor and those he rallies around him if you want to go where others cannot and receive information hidden to most. In fact, much of the national, state, and local information gathered without the benefit of such alliances is not complete. Pastors and their recruits can knock on doors and be welcomed into any home, they can ask questions and get complete, factual answers. They can measure household smoke levels and find out what food people are eating, inspect for lead paint, record who is HIV-positive, and much more.

Respect and recognition of those who have helped is critical. Publicly acknowledge those who have helped at meetings, in reports, books, articles, and with the press. Those who helped may not be seeking a pat on the back, but they are not looking for a slap in the face either. There is nothing worse than one of those assistants picking up documents and seeing the names of the institutions, researchers, and community health workers and not seeing theirs.

The minister normally opens the doors of the community for the institution to poke, prod, prove, or disprove. In a true partnership, the doors are open both ways. Invite the minister or other community leaders to ask questions and learn from the institution. Give them opportunities to teach others within the institution, including students and coworkers. In showing fairness and equality, allow the guest lecturers or teachers, if they qualify based upon their education and experience, to issue grades. Otherwise, the students and others within the organization do not take the teacher or subject matter seriously. Providing the opportunity is not enough; validation is necessary.

Where possible include the minister as a principal or coprincipal investigator on the grant, especially if contact and assistance occurred before submitting the grant and if institutions expect the minister to continue to help upon funding. When the minister or other community assistants speak at conferences, teach classes, or do work for which institutions pay other professionals, compensate them accordingly. Give them the proper honorarium or expense reimbursement. It is insulting to give something for nothing when others are being paid. Many other components of developing a true partnership will become apparent as the details of the relationship are worked out.

Done properly, the institution can gain an advocate for life in the clergy and the people helped. The voices of the people ring much louder and are sounder than those of critics. Those voices of praise help to establish and sustain relationships within the community and even other communities for future projects. Do keep in mind that most churches and pastors belong to regional and national groups, so a positive interaction locally can lead to national recognition and acceptance in other inner-city communities.

Overall, the ultimate goal and measure of success is when the partners no longer look at each other as just partners, but as part of a single community health team with a long-term objective. Benefiting the community should be the focus of all workers involved.

Community Relations

Forming an alliance based on equality creates significant levels of credibility and acceptance, but that still is not enough. Positive and well-grounded community relations are essential to the success of any program or research activity with the inner city. While many African Americans are by nature very open and accepting, assuring them of the value of the work requires a conscious community-relations effort before, during, and even after the project has ended. Without this outreach component, there is still a risk of nonacceptance, skepticism, and limited participation, all of which can affect the ease of conducting work, interacting with individuals, the timeliness of obtaining the desired outcome, and the overall success and integrity of the work.

Frankly, even with a free program to prevent heart attacks, people are not going to flock to it because they want to know if there is a catch, what the institution is gaining, and what they or the community is giving up. They raise these questions because they have experienced, perceived, or have heard about a history of being deceived, misunderstood, and used by white Americans and "the system." However, they also want to be included in what is going on around them. So, cautiously, they may question just why volunteers would come into their community and do a project with no strings attached.

The truth is that the institution and its workers do gain something, whether it is research data, case studies, or other information. The researchers write books, appear on television, and advance their careers largely because of the support and cooperation of the community. The community knows the institution has something to gain and ultimately they will see it in different forms. This is why service components that benefit the community beyond the programmatic aspects of the project are important. Institutions must think out and incorporate these service components before approaching the community. Additionally, the institution must remain flexible enough to make changes after coming into the community and assessing needs.

Again, use the church as a key conduit to the community, while not ignoring other sources as well. Bypassing the church, the center of the African American community, will eventually create problems for community health workers individually and institutions as a whole because there will be no stamp of approval, no assurances or reassurances, and no checks and balances. The community may assume that the project is self-centered, thus affecting the outcome. The church is not going to dilute the efforts of any organization that can legitimately help. On the contrary, the church adds legitimacy as well as relevance and effectiveness. Beyond the functional components of typical community-relations programs, the very nature of health-related projects within inner cities requires specific planning and programmatic incorporation in three general areas: cultural understanding, community involvement, and timing. Cultural understanding comes through community involvement, so those two areas are addressable jointly. Knowing the right time to launch the program is the result of successfully addressing the first two areas.

Reading a couple of books, speaking with African American colleagues, or watching a couple of "culturally correct" movies does not reveal the cultural dynamics of the chosen community. The most detrimental mistake that can ground the program before it even takes off is launching it without understanding and appreciating the culture of the targeted people or place. Human nature instills a false feeling in most people that, with a little bit of knowledge, they know what is best. Of course, this is narrow-minded thinking and hinders any type of interpersonal interaction.

No one knows everything, and nor does the church. Still, the church and its leader can help. Find out what it will take to accomplish the institution's aims. Be prepared to accept new ideas. Ask what will offend the community, from the most simple infringements to those that are complex. For example, going into the community with a brochure featuring only pictures of white people sends the message that the program or the illness only concerns whites. Institutions can avoid these types of problems easily, but the potential damage could take months to overcome. In this case, proactive steps include letting church representatives look at existing materials and asking for help in producing new materials. Community relations works in both directions, so consult with people who can eliminate unintentional trouble.

Although the church can be of great assistance, it is necessary to obtain information firsthand by personally interacting with the community. Opportunities for community interaction include the following: attending church services and activities; participating in community events; patronizing businesses, such as restaurants and convenience stores; visiting local libraries; offering training to the church and community members; giving technical, physical, and financial assistance; providing scholarships and internships; developing mentoring programs; and conducting seminars. Every community is different and has its own needs, so look for other available opportunities to create a positive, interaction with all members of the community, not just the community leaders.

Participation in and sponsorship of such activities are excellent opportunities to learn about the individuals who make up the community. A college degree or vast research resources do not provide a sense of the cultural pulse of the community. These resources may seem to provide the necessary knowledge, but the reality is that the institution and its designated workers are probably not from that particular environment. Although there may be a burning desire to be helpful, it does not always work out that way because of a lack of preparation. There is an old proverb that takes place in a flood: A frog was hopping from place to place trying to avoid being covered by the water. A bird came down, picked the frog up, and placed it in a tree. As the water continued to rise, the bird thought it had done the frog a big favor and expected the frog to be thankful. However, the frog replied that being in the tree would kill it and that its chances for survival were better in the water. In effect, the frog did not respond to the "good deed" the way the bird anticipated.

Members of research and community health teams sometimes receive this type of response. Coming into the community with a "savior" mentality does not always work because the residents are already surviving. Raising their survival level is another issue. Without knowing what mode of survival people are in, it is hard to know where and how to begin, how far to go, what is realistic, and what is acceptable. Being open and adapting nonjudgmentally to the ways of the community and its residents is essential. For example, there are differences in the ways that white and African Americans raise their children. Accordingly, there are aspects of parenting that are acceptable and not acceptable to both groups. This does not mean that either parents are not good parents. Certainly, parenting skills can be shared with anyone, but the acceptance and use of those shared skills are contingent upon understanding the differences in environment and what constitutes a family, among other considerations. An African American family is not a "typical" family. Instead, aunts raise nieces, grandparents raise grandchildren, daughters care for grandparents, and neighbors take care of neighbors. African Americans frown upon nursing homes and will turn to them as the absolute last resort. There are obvious differences in dress and language among the races, but these should not be judged critically. Instead, there must be an acknowledgment of lifestyle and cultural differences, but these do not make any group more or less than the other. Americans accept differences between themselves and other nationalities more readily than they do among each other.

It takes time to break barriers, build bridges, and gain a comfort level with and among the community. Do not expect to start a program immediately. It takes time to know the church, its pastor, community organizations and leaders, and cultural dynamics to carry out the program at the highest level of acceptance and effectiveness possible. Through interaction and understanding, changes may be required to the research instrument and the methodology or the service component may need defining or redefining. It may be clear by the response that it is the appropriate time to move ahead. But if there is any doubt, ask the minister and any other community leader who can test the waters to avoid the mistake the bird made with the frog.

Communications

While the bird and the frog clearly had difficulties understanding where the other was "coming from," it would have been just as difficult had they attempted to communicate with each other using their own language and communication styles. Likewise, it is important to adapt verbal and written communications to reach inner-city residents, from the community leader to the drug-addicted resident.

One of the first, but perhaps most important, lessons is that the African American community communicates differently than institutions. Communication is less formal and time-consuming and more action-oriented. The community reacts to verbal communications more than meetings and letters. Long letters often go unread after the first paragraph or two, not because people cannot read, but because they do not have the time and it simply is not the way information is generally transmitted within the community. Communicating through churches or throughout the community does not require a special meeting or effort that takes time that many people do not have. It is not unusual for residents of the community to obtain information from others while walking down the street, at the barber shop, in the grocery store, or during church. These are places of congregation and communication in the inner city. And the most prevalent way to release that information is through the pulpit. The church is the primary source and the preacher is the primary communicator.

Usually, if the information is important to the individual he will make a mental note or will jot it down on a piece of paper. When meeting with a minister or a community resident or leader, if that person takes the time to write something down then it is clearly important to them. However, do not be offended if ministers or others come to meetings without pencils and paper. They happen to be good listeners and will remember what needs to be acted upon and when, but only if it is important to them. If you make a promise to get back in touch with someone within a given time, do so. African Americans hold promises dear. Even if the initial response is not what you expected, be courteous and place a call or write a note. Showing a change of mind will not make it impossible to work with the community in the future. What it shows is respect and concern. A lack of follow-through or response, on the other hand, is perceived often as a lack of seriousness and a desire just to take from the community. Even if this particular project does not go through, since some inroads have been made, keep communication channels open for future projects by remaining involved in the community. Lend technical abilities and skills in other areas or provide assistance through other efforts.

When the project advances, the community health worker has to find the best ways to communicate to the targeted audience and obtain the required feedback. It is easy to make mistakes just through style of listening or body language. If a person feels that he or she is not being listened to, communication and trust can easily break down. Within the African American community, once a person or group decides to open up and share information, that line of communication can close very quickly if the information shared is not taken seriously. Listen actively, carefully, and respectfully.

Body language and verbal expressions are used to gauge interest, sincerity, respect, and honesty. In African American homes, a mother will often say to a child, "let me look in your eyes to see if you are telling the truth." Mannerisms and expressions show more than words can express. People can use words to be untruthful, but they cannot hide their true feelings.

African Americans take seriously the phrases "the truth shall make you free" and "honesty is next to godliness." Whatever the truth is, know it and lay it out up front. It is worse if some untruth or partial story creates the impression of a lie. Lying is considered a major sin or crime among African Americans and is not easily forgiven or forgotten. A lie sets back progress, ends cooperation, shuts down programs, and deters future projects by any other organization.

Simply knowing how to approach a person and what to say or not to say is critical to having a positive and productive communication experience. Learn how to approach a person and be invited into their home by finding out which phrases or words to use or avoid. On the other hand, trying to imitate others is the "worst" form of flattery. Recognizing the differences in communication and expression and working within the existing network is the best solution, and this effort must extend beyond the fieldworkers and into the larger institution. For example, if an individual goes to the emergency room of a hospital and is mistreated, in the future that bad experience is associated with anything to do with the entire institution. It becomes hard to work with that individual or with anyone in the community who hears about the experience.

The clergy can help the institution by serving as trainers, mediators, and translators. Actually, they work on behalf of both the institution and the community. They train both in how to work with each other and solve conflicts or misunderstandings, and they convey and interpret what is said and what is meant. The clergy bridges the gap in communication styles and skills. An effective use of the clergy is to invite them into the institution to conduct seminars, role playing, and training before fieldwork begins. What they can share is invaluable.

The relationship between the clergy, community, and institution is like a marriage; notably, one of the first things that go wrong in marriages is a failure to communicate effectively. From that come arguments, misunderstandings, and divorce. If the partnership is going to flourish, there must be open and frequent communication throughout the relationship. Today's electronic advances offer numerous opportunities to communicate or touch base, every day if necessary. And as in marriage, some counseling in advance of forming the union is beneficial to all. This "all" includes the institution and its workers, the clergy, and community residents.

CHAPTER FOUR

Finding and Securing Funding

REGARDLESS OF THE CITY, situation, or solution, the one common thread for everyone who wants to work toward solving the problem is a problem itself: obtaining funding. I have always taken the attitude that what God expects of us in our display of belief in Him is that we "Walk by faith and not by sight." We may not see the funds we need right away, but if we remain faithful, patient, and determined, everything will work out. At the same time, though, we have to understand the process of seeking funds and learn how we can have the best possible chance of obtaining them.

It is fundamental to have a firm understanding of how grants work. Overall, they are given with the expectation of getting something in return, for example, research data, medical results, or a change in attitudes and behavior. The grant is not a gift. It is money used for something the funding source needs. Furthermore, each foundation makes funding decisions based upon a particular agenda. It could be to influence local or national policies, to change public opinion on an issue, or to align themselves with a particular target market. Many are not inclined to fund the extension of programs run elsewhere. Some are interested in local versus national outcomes, while others want to pursue innovative and creative start-up projects. Some will fund research and others will not. The key is finding a funding source with the same interests and mission as your church or organization, and then showing how, with their funding, you can help them meet their goals. Corporate donations are also made in self-interest. Usually the money is designated for areas where the corporation has a presence and for issues that the corporation has

identified to position itself positively among the public, its employees, and possibly its investors. Other funding sources include local
and state health departments, state bond bills, community development block grants, the U.S. Department of Health and Human
Services, and the National Institutes of Health.

Too Many Needs, Too Few Dollars

From the onset you have to assess the many diverse needs of the
community and decide which one you and your church or organization plan on tackling. If you try to solve too many problems at
once you will not solve any, and will ultimately create more problems because you have made promises or built up expectations that
you cannot meet. Also, keep in mind that if you gain a reputation
for not following through on projects, you will have trouble con-
vincing an organization to partner with you or provide funding in
the future. The needs are many, but it is important that you satisfy
them one or two at a time. If you have a partner, have partnered
before, or have universities or hospitals in your area, use them as a
resource in the process of gathering information and making decisions about feasible projects. In assessing the possibilities, be realistic about what you think you, with appropriate backing, can accomplish. We often take on more than we can handle because many of
our inner-city problems seem to be "larger than life." You have to
remember that these problems did not occur overnight, nor can they
be solved quickly or by you alone. However, once you have identified the issue or problem you want to address and have the support
of the church, think about what you can do until you receive funding—and what you can do if you do not. Obviously, funding and
partnering is the desired outcome, but every project simply will not
have that level of support. When identifying the issue and rallying
the support of the congregation and others, you have to be prepared
to take some type of action with or without the assistance of an outside source. Otherwise you lose credibility among the community

and especially those who would have been helped by your project. These people are usually people who have been disappointed too often already. Helping a few is better than disappointing many.

Consider the changes to and impact on the church or organization should the grant request be met. Some issues to address include:

1. What will be the immediate resources and changes required of the congregation, such as buses and vans or alterations to the physical building?
2. What changes to your schedule will be necessary and will your congregation accept these changes?
3. What will be the short- and long-term financial and operational consequences?
4. Will the project change the focus, mission, or character of the church?
5. Will the funding of the project affect funding from other sources for different projects?

Other questions should be raised about the project, the funding source, and the organization seeking funding. Do not be blindsided or underestimate the changes, from the positive to the challenging, that funding can cause. The best thing is to be prepared for just about anything. Make up a couple of possible scenarios or situations and determine how they would be handled.

In identifying the problem to be addressed, you have to be creative and selective. You have to conduct research. No organization is going to fund what five other groups have already done in the community. The need has to be compelling and growing, sometimes untouched, local yet with national significance, and able to be verified. How many people are affected now? Will it affect more in the future? Will it have long-term effects on their lives? If a program is carried out, is it possible to measure results? How long will it take before being able to measure and report the results? These are just some of the questions you should ask about any proposed project because these are the same ones that any funding source will want answers to as well. Remember that the funding source is results-driven and wants to see a "return" on their money through positive outcomes, new community models, and the like. They are not just giving the money to serve your community. They are trying to fund and develop programs that they can transfer to other cities and that can be used to teach instructors, students, community health workers, and community leaders. Recognize that you alone will not own this project. If successfully carried out, it will be used repeatedly elsewhere.

The best way to identify and determine the cause for which you will seek funding is to get outside the church and talk to people other than those in the congregation. Go to the streets and knock on doors and assess what is or is not taking place in your community. You might be surprised to learn that there is a high incidence of ringworm or that most of the children have never had a hearing test or eye exam. Or, you may find more serious problems such as widespread high blood pressure or heart disease where people are not seeking or receiving the appropriate care. You might decide to focus on preventive care, to set up roving clinics for vision and hearing testing, or to begin a program to teach people how to reduce their blood pressure. Before deciding definitively what to do, check to see if other resources are available nearby that people simply have not taken advantage of, and investigate whether local hospitals and institutions might be a resource based upon their focus and interests. If you have personal contacts at local institutions or know others who do, learn about current research and training activities. You might find a partner or funding resource simply by expressing an interest and asking a couple of questions. Realistically, this does not happen very often, but when you see a community and its people hurting, it is always worth a try.

Funding Sources

There are many sources for obtaining funding, but you have to seek them out. Because of the number of requests they receive, they certainly will not come looking for you and your organization. Proactive research to identify potential funding sources takes time and has to be done systematically. You may not have time to do it yourself and will have to delegate it to another. A word of caution if you do: make sure the person is committed, conscientious, capable, and above all willing to put the necessary time into the project. Many organizations hire someone to find the potential grantors as well as write the proposals and complete applications.

In researching foundations or other organizations to request funding, first check your local library for books that identify funding sources. These books are normally found in the reference section, and since often you cannot check them out you may want to go to your local bookstore and purchase a couple of books. Also, do not overlook online computer services or conducting your own search on the Internet. During this process, you will find you need to narrow your search by identifying the type of funding source you are seeking. You certainly do not want nor will it be possible or necessary to contact every potential funding source. You have to screen and qualify them, just as they will do the same with your proposal or application. What you should consider first is the type of funding, such as whether the organization gives matching funds or loans. Often organizations apply for funds without realizing the full scope of the requirements, which can entail raising matching funds or meeting certain performance requirements. You have to approach the organization with attention to its funding methods as well as its interests. Necessary information includes the geographic preference for funding, special priorities and interests, project and applicant type preferences, recent grantees, if any projects in your geographic area or with similar focus have been funded, and the average amount of the funding.

Obtaining this information does take quite a bit of time. Be aware, though, that information is always changing and chances are that by the time you finish some information will be outdated. Also, you may receive information by telephone or in writing and find later that the requirements, deadlines, or another important detail have changed. Because of the number of people who make inquiries and the number of applicants, there is no way that the foundation can let everyone know. Further, the foundation can change their published requirements anytime, without being accountable to you or to anyone else. Therefore, try to establish and maintain direct contact to stay abreast of new staff, shifts in priorities, changes in guidelines, or special opportunities. If possible, schedule a personal visit in an attempt to establish a relationship or at least name and face recognition. After the research is conducted, you should have a list of no more than 10 possible contacts, if that many. If you have more, then you need to pare the list down even further. However, once you see what they require it is unlikely that you will plan to submit applications or proposals to even five sources.

While every foundation, corporation, or other funding source has its own individual application forms, there are some basic, common questions that you need to be prepared to answer. Having short, clear, and concise answers ready are key to the ease in which you can probably complete applications, answer questions during interviews, and explain the project and the funding need to others. The following questions are some of the ones for which you should have responses:

1. What is the project?
2. Who is/are the applicant(s)?
3. How will the applicant(s) be able to conduct or help with conducting the project?
4. What, if any, special talents, experiences, etc., does the applicant(s) bring to the project?
5. Who are the beneficiaries of the project?
6. What are the short and long-term benefits of the project?
7. What are the project's initial and ongoing costs?
8. Will the applicant(s) be able to contribute monetarily to the funding or contribute in other ways, either initially or eventually?

9. Who will do the work?

10. Is there a location for the work to take place?

11. What is expected of the funding source beyond funds?

12. Who else, individuals or other funding sources, is supporting this project?

13. Who can be contacted for references?

14. What is the financial condition of your organization?

15. Do you have audited statements?

16. How is your organization structured?

17. Have you worked with foundations or corporations previously?

18. Have you applied previously, successfully or unsuccessfully, for funds for this project or other projects?

19. What other projects do you currently or have you previously operated?

20. Why is it important to support and fund this project?

Once you have responses to these questions, let someone with grant-writing or grant-giving experience look at them. If possible, have at least two experts review the questions and answers and then compare their comments and make whatever changes are appropriate. Be sure to keep your final questions and answers in a safe place and make duplicate copies, as you and others will be referring to these frequently.

Now that you have identified the foundations and are prepared to write your proposal, it is almost time to get down to work. However, there are several other things you need to consider to give your proposal an edge over the others. Think about how the particular foundation can benefit from providing funding for the project. After all, funders are in search of ways and means, such as your group, to deal with visible community problems or their funding priorities. Your goal should be to position your organization or church as the best and right vehicle to address a particular issue. There are other organizations and churches that may be vying for the same funds, so take a good look at what your organization has to offer. Identify what is unique about it, where progress has been made, what projects have been successfully completed, if projects have longevity or have served many people or a population rarely served, if there is something that your church was first to do. Just like television commercials, the message is always sprinkled with why a particular product is different or better. Now is the time to brag a little. These bragging points may be just what will separate your proposal and subsequent consideration from others. Consider this action as helping the funding source sift through the applications and select those for further consideration, including, of course, your proposal.

While writing your proposal, keep in mind that the person reading it probably has hundreds of requests to read, along with other job responsibilities. Words of advice: Keep it Short and Simple. Do not feel that you have to use large, impressive words to show your vocabulary skills. Make sure the writing is easy to read and understandable. Even if you have to use technical terms, be sure to include a definition of the terms and try to use them sparingly, especially if you think the reader may not be familiar with the terms. Additionally, give several pages of the proposal to someone else to read and get their opinion on the writing. After one reading, ask them about what they read. If they have difficulties understanding it, you may need to adjust your copy. Another consideration, especially to help the busy reader, is to prepare a table of contents and a summary of your proposal. The summary will give the reader a quick tool to assess the merit of your request and it gives you the opportunity to put your strongest, most impressive points first. Think about ways to present or package your proposal so that it appeals visually to the reader. However, make sure that there are no application rules prohibiting any of your packaging ideas. Moreover, you do not want the packaging to distract from the proposal or make it any longer. Some considerations are the use of colored paper, borders, binding, colored ink, specialty papers, and photographs, among other enhancement ideas.

Before submitting the proposal, do not hesitate to use whatever contacts you have to lobby for support, provide advice, give references, and to help in other ways. As long as you are not doing anything unethical, there is nothing wrong with getting some help. Furthermore, the foundation will still make its choice based upon the standard set and there may be two or more organizations besides yours that are qualified. After completing the proposal and submitting it for review, do not be afraid or hesitant to call to make sure they received it and to track the status of the awarding process. Ask specifically when you should call, the best time of day, and if you should ask for a specific person. If you call and ask whether you should call or write, the person will likely say to write rather than call them, but assume you can call unless told otherwise. If handled properly, this is just another technique of setting yourself and your proposal apart and above the rest. Being proactive and following up shows the organization the type of standards they can expect when dealing with you and your church or organization.

The Upside and Downside

Obtaining funding is not without its ups and downs. You should be aware of and anticipate both. The benefits of receiving outside funds may find include:

1. It can help to replace competition with coordination and unity in the planning, promotion, and implementation of programs and in fundraising among the denominations and community groups.

2. It may influence a spirit of unity and outreach among other churches or community groups, or even within the church or community group itself.

3. It can provide freedom from an ongoing appeal to the same people and organizations for funds for different causes, which some-

times causes confusion and a deliberate determination not to give.

4. Funding can provide steady, reliable support and end the cycle of indebtedness, thus making growth and expansion possible.

5. It provides a built-in system of financial checks and balances and accountability.

6. It often prompts long-range planning instead of constant preoccupation with ever-present survival issues.

On the downside, some drawbacks caused by outside funding may include the following:

1. An overemphasis on the program that is being funded, like the new kid on the block, may be at the expense of other existing programs that are just as important.

2. The project may be perceived as impersonal because the institutions or companies involved are big.

3. There will be times when responses and reactions are not as quick as expected, which can lead to a perception of being taken for granted.

4. Because there is a lot to know about the funding source and its requirements, some applicants do not take the time to learn what is necessary. As a result, many problems can arise that impact trust and confidence.

5. Over-protectiveness and ownership can make the program budget a tug-of-war, with nothing accomplished and making change very difficult.

6. The tendency to treat reporting requirements too lightly, which often causes unnecessary conflict or suspicion.

These few strengths and weaknesses described can grow out of the personalities, backgrounds, expectations, and experiences of the people involved. They will mirror the levels of commitment and trust, the degree of unity, and the participants' practices and priorities. Everyone must remember that the resultant project belongs to everyone, not just one group, and that probably not everyone will be satisfied with how the money is allocated or what is or is not included. With the proper structure, however, it will reflect the consensus of the majority.

Keeping the Funds Flowing

While there is no guarantee that your project will continue to receive long-term funding, some measures help to ensure that the partners' relationship is such that the funding source would feel confident in continuing support. While these points may seem simplistic and are things you probably would do anyway, realize that the funding source places a lot more importance and significance on these than you think, especially if it is not in the same city where you are located. Share information regularly, and in a consistent format, about the project's success in reaching its goals, keeping accurate documentation of services, training, and outreach, and identifying areas where change is needed to avoid problems. Report benefits and outcomes that go beyond what was originally expected, such as the provision of jobs and learning opportunities among community residents, the ability to get information to traditionally hard-to-reach members of the community, community involvement and ownership, and crossing cultural barriers. Follow all financial reporting and spending requirements strictly and without any deviation. If you do not have someone within the congregation or group who can handle financial management, take the time and money to find someone even before you begin to receive funds. The management of the funds is an area that they will scrutinize during the project and will also be used to evaluate the possibility of funding at another time. As in the Bible, God is not going to give you more if you cannot handle a little. The same applies in dealing with your funding source.

Seek opportunities for the funding source to gain recognition within the community, including as part of any local, regional, or national speaking engagements, seminars, and media coverage. Involve representatives of the funding source in as much of the project as possible so they can see their dollars at work rather than only read a report. Give them opportunities to meet and speak to representatives of the community, the population served, and the congregation. Do not make them a silent partner in the project. Another consideration is always to stay on top of the funding source's interest and look for additional opportunities in the community. Present those opportunities and any other ideas you have throughout the relationship. Do not wait to share your thoughts until the funding source asks all interested groups to submit proposals. Try to both encourage expansion of the existing project and pursue other projects. With your partner, sit down and discuss jointly pursuing funding for mutually interesting projects and programs. A collaborative effort from the onset may produce even greater results for all parties. Above all, what is most important is to try to stay ahead of your competition as much as possible to get a fair share of the dollars available.

Self-Sufficiency

Funding can bring ideas to life, add strength, and build excitement. It is the backbone of most community-based programs. But there is a need to use other support systems as well, because rejection is a reality. Unfortunately, there will not always be enough funds from a foundation, and sometimes no funds at all. You cannot wait and let your programs come to a screeching halt because the funding source is no longer available. Do not set yourself or your group up by forgetting how it used to be, because things can easily revert to how they were. Funding is never permanently assured; it must be sought after and renewed continuously. Even when beginning to seek funds, start an independent process of establishing your own source of financial support. This will demonstrate your organization's seriousness and commitment to dealing with the problem or providing the necessary service to the community. Some ways of raising money include special offerings at church, individual designated gifts, earned income from selling materials, speaking, or training, and even the development of your own endowment fund.

Benefitting From Rejection

Sometimes your competition simply can better provide what the funding source is seeking than you can at this time. In short, you might not get the money. Well, this will not be the first time or the last, but learning as much as you can from the rejection will move you closer to receiving a positive response to your request. Call or write the funding source and ask for specific reasons why they did not fund your proposal and what you can do in the future to have a better chance. With this information you will be more prepared and can approach the funding source again, and successfully. Also, find out what churches, partnerships, or community organizations did receive funding. Examine their programs to see what they offer and compare them to your organization. What does their program offer that yours did not? What are the differences and similarities between your organization and the others? When you prepare your next proposal, perhaps focus on including or highlighting comparable programmatic services and organizational similarities. Rejection will take you back into the realm of research, but in applying what you have learned to your next proposal, you will gain even stronger prospects for future funding.

CHAPTER FIVE

Marketing the Message

As SHOWN BY THE PROGRAM described in Chapter Three, special emphasis must be placed on how to "spread the word." Of great importance is the church and its partner identifying the most effective means of communicating with the intended audience. Several creative methods are described in this chapter; these were prepared by churches, however, there are many ways that the partner can get the message out to the target audience. These can include setting up displays in public places, passing out premium items imprinted with information, conducting contests and other participatory activities, transit and billboard advertising, videos, slide shows, radio commercials, and signs and flyers at community gathering locations.

While conversation is the primary method of sharing general information among inner-city residents, some instructions or details simply cannot be passed along by word-of-mouth and churches and their partners will have to go beyond the typical. For example, instead of producing a basic booklet on diabetes, compile a cookbook for diabetics or a shopper's guide to food substitutes. Consider creating a "healthy habits" coloring book for children to address issues such as cleanliness, the spreading of germs, good eating habits, or proper dental hygiene. Community health campaigns have to be creative in deciding how to present information and incorporate it into acceptable and useful formats.

Marketing for awareness and program involvement within the inner city requires at a minimum a concerted grassroots effort that goes hand-in-hand with establishing a relationship with the clergy and developing community relations. Knowing that communication among residents tends to be informal and brief, appropriate and effective marketing and advertising actions have the same characteristics. While a range of marketing and advertising techniques should be considered, the most effective for program participation is door-to-door, neighborhood canvassing. The advantage of going door-to-door with church partners or having the church handle it altogether is that the clergy and church representatives have access that outsiders do not possess. People are not going to open their doors for just anyone. They know the churches in the neighborhood, the preachers, and the congregation. They come to the church for services and assistance and they anticipate representatives coming to them at some point. When the canvassers work in the neighborhood, they must wear something identifiable such as a hat, T-shirt, or jacket with the project logo. Without this form of visible identification, some doors will not open.

Once those doors are opened to receive a church representative, the visit often has a social aspect that goes beyond simply giving or taking information. Many people are glad to have company, they may be elderly or homebound or they simply need someone with whom to talk. Anyone participating in door-to-door canvassing has to be flexible enough to spend anywhere from five minutes to an hour for visits. If someone wants to talk, it is important to listen even if the conversation is not about the research project or service offering. It is important to be a good listener as these homes will more than likely be visited again. When going door-to-door, churches have found it effective to present more than one program or service to the resident. This provides an opportunity to take a holistic approach to the needs of the person and household. In addition, it eliminates the perception that the visitor is concerned with just one issue, that of the project or program. Canvassing is not limited to going to homes. Have representatives pass out literature or talk with people on street corners or in front of high-traffic locations like grocery stores. All canvassing methods provide the marketing opportunity to encourage people to come to events and visit program or service sites. Other methods, while simple, will help to recruit volunteers, promote meetings and events, and publicize program locations and hours of operation. These simple methods include placing posters, flyers, and brochures on bulletin boards in churches, schools, libraries, and retail and service locations. Program information can be conveyed on church fans, Sunday bulletins, newsletters, mailers, and programs for church events. And the information will continue to spread by word of mouth among community residents. Knowing this, it is important for community health workers to communicate information as clearly and thoroughly as possible, because it will be passed on verbally.

Overall, the grassroots marketing and advertising approach is effective; however, it is not completely accepted by the clergy. Why? Because it cannot compete with the marketing and advertising presence of corporations, associations, and other entities. Some believe that if they had the same advertising dollars of cigarette and alcoholic beverage companies, they could make major changes in the overall health of the community through messages on prevention and care. The advertising that most inner-city residents see, particularly on billboards and buses in their neighborhoods, promotes the ills of the community and essentially what its leaders are trying to eliminate. Newborn babies are brought into homes smelling cigarette smoke, when they begin to see colors they see billboards featuring cigarettes, and as they get older they see enticing ads in magazines. These messages surround them during their impressionable years, a time when they want acceptance and succumb to peer pressure. Ironically, smoking on buses is illegal, yet the outside of the vehicles are covered with ads promoting cigarettes. What a contradiction and a shame. The same advertising space could show positive pictures of healthy people and provide messages about good health practices.

The money that is available for advertising is simply not enough. In the case of money received from the federal government, the $100,000 for the total project becomes $50,000 at the state level. Once it reaches the city, it drops to $25,000. Finally, when it reaches the community or activity for which it was originally intended, only $10,000 is left. This funding allocation process is upside down. If the $100,000 was placed directly into the community there would be greater results. Many grants for community projects do not include funds for advertising, or restrict marketing efforts to the grassroots approach. Now, churches challenge institutions to include advertising in grant requests or to enhance the grant with funds designated for advertising.

At the community level, there is a need for complete marketing and advertising campaigns that are geographically focused within the area where the planned program or service is to take place. Since many residents of these inner-city areas watch television and listen to urban contemporary or Christian radio, broadcast media buys are necessary. The success of the media buy depends on incorporating the insights of clergy or African Americans who are aware of the dynamics of the inner city into the development of marketing materials and advertisements. Often advertising efforts are wasted because the ads were produced by whites or out-of-touch African Americans who simply do not know what reaches inner-city residents. They do not know what to say and how it should be said. In this instance, consult with the clergy and use them and their representatives for focus groups and as advisors. The benefit to consulting with the church is that the pastor and congregation know the real issues and can anticipate problems. For example, while teen pregnancy is a problem, many religious leaders knew the use of the contraceptive Norplant was not the solution. They complained not just from a religious standpoint, but also from a health-concern platform. They knew that Norplant was not a safe product to use among a population with a history of high blood pressure and strokes. The insight of the ministers was cast aside. There are now many lawsuits because of the use of Norplant among African Americans. While this controversy did not focus on advertising, it clearly shows the importance of speaking with and heeding the advice of the clergy.

When developing marketing and advertising strategies, most

members of the clergy would advise against telephone surveys because more accurate and complete information comes through face-to-face meetings. Workshops, health fairs, and seminars are common ways to share and receive information among the African American community. These should be kept brief but informative, with time for questions and answers. Simple information can be gathered during canvassing; however, most people are not willing to stop what they are doing in their homes to answer lengthy questionnaires. If they do, they may not spend the time to think through each question thoroughly as they just want to complete the information and get back to what they were doing. Reserve detailed questionnaires for when people come to a program office, church, or another location. At that point, they have time to talk and are willing to share information. Of course, the questionnaire must be developed with consideration for the neighborhood culture, the education level of the residents, the age of the targeted interviewees, and other demographic requirements. Again, consult with the clergy on the questionnaire. They know how to word questions to elicit a response and can encourage participation from and beyond the pulpit.

Spreading the Word

Through thoughtful collaboration between the partners and extensive interaction with the community, the project can discover the best means of getting the message out to its targeted audience. The following examples are drawn from actual programs and show how information can be effectively presented at different stages of the project. A review of these will help you to determine what will work best in your community or to enhance what your church or institution may be doing already.

Slide Shows

Concise slide shows can be very useful introductions to explain the nature of the project and to solicit the support necessary. Heart,

Body, and Soul, a program developed by the Baltimore-based Clergy United For the Renewal of East Baltimore (CURE), started with no funds and grew to include smoking cessation programs in 22 churches, blood pressure training and referrals, CPR training, training in breast cancer detection, and cholesterol and nutritional screening programs. As a result of this one-of-a-kind program, a health services cost review commission illness prevention program was developed that allows the hospital to increase rates by a fraction of a penny per admission and to put funds back into prevention programs for the community.

CURE developed a slide show presentation to introduce the program and the institutional partner, Johns Hopkins Academic Health Center, to the community. The show addressed the issues that were most likely to concern the residents and influence their support for and participation in the project, including:

1. What is CURE and what is Heart, Body, and Soul?
2. What will the partners provide?
3. Why do we need a Heart, Body, and Soul Project? What are the health problems affecting our community?
4. How will the project help solve these problems?
5. Why are churches involved?
6. What is the long-term goal?
7. Why do we need to work together?
8. What exactly will this project offer the community?
9. How can my church be involved?

Fact Sheets

With information provided by medical authorities, an East Baltimore ministry developed a series of informational sheets on topics such as diabetes, vision, substance abuse, and asthma. These materials are inexpensive yet informative tools for marketing and awareness among residents and volunteers. The Garden of Prayer's Health Ministries produced a fact sheet "Sounding the Trumpet of Good Health About Diabetes!" that began with a message from the minister, citing Hosea 4:6, Our People Will Perish Because of a Lack of Knowledge. The fact sheet provided specific information on diabetes and how it affects African Americans, including these sample passages:

"The Garden of Prayer Baptist Church believes in a holistic ministry including the Spirit, Soul, and Body. Our members and officers believe in promoting healthy lifestyles in our community. It is our desire and intention to spread the gospel of good health throughout the world. So, join with us in sounding the trumpet of good health."

"Diabetes, with its serious complications, is estimated to affect more than 12 million Americans, half of whom are totally unaware that they have the illness. This incurable disease is caused by the body's failure to produce or properly use insulin, a hormone that is needed by the human body to convert sugar, starches, and other foods into the energy required for daily life. Diabetes often leads to serious complications involving nearly every tissue of the body."

"Diabetes is a major risk factor for: kidney disease; retinopathy/blindness; peripheral vascular disease (ulcers that lead to amputations); coronary heart disease; cerebrovascular disease."

"Prevalence Among African Americans: African Americans and Hispanics represent 22% of all people with diabetes. The rate of Type II Diabetes is 33% higher among African Americans and 300% higher among Hispanics than white Americans. African Americans with Type II Diabetes have mortality rates twice that of whites. Diabetic Nephropathy (End-Stage Renal Disease) is three times higher among African Americans than whites. African American women older than 54 have diabetes 1.5 times more than African American men."

"Risk Factors: female gender; family history; children born to mothers older than 35; obesity." "Prevention Strategies: proper diet; weight reduction; improved education and self-management skills; regular eye and physical exams."

Handouts can also be used to share tips or advice, for example, to reach the person who is attempting to stop smoking as well as those who are assisting or serving as the support base. These can be presented in an accessible format yet still offer inspiration to the reader, as shown in this excerpt from *One Day at A Time, For Personal Guidance in Quitting Smoking,* published by the Clergy United for the Renewal of East Baltimore:

"Stop smoking tip: Learn to relax. When life is hard and you want to smoke, sit down in a quiet place. Close your eyes, and take a few deep breaths. As you do, talk gently to yourself in a quiet and calm way and you will begin to feel the calm spread through your body. Let God help you feel at peace. When you feel calmer, picture yourself throwing all of your cigarettes away. Keep practicing."

Readings: Psalms 70:1: "Make haste, O God, to deliver me! Make haste to help me, O Lord!" Psalm 70:5: "But I am poor and needy; make haste unto me O God: thou art my help and deliverer; O Lord make no tarrying." Matthew 2:28: "Come unto me all you who labor and are heavy laden, and I will give you rest." Matthew 2:29: "Take my yoke upon you and learn of me; for I am meek and lowly in heart; and ye shall find rest unto your souls." Matthew 2:20: "For my yoke is easy, and my burden is light."

"If we feel nobody understands, remember God understands. Sometimes I feel that nobody understands how hard it is to stop smoking. I feel that I am struggling all alone and something seems to be missing. I may even feel sorry for myself. I start to think one cigarette will not hurt me. I may tell myself that I miss smoking so much that I do not have the will to fight. Worst of all, I feel no one is there to help me, no one cares or understands how truly hard it is to quit smoking. I need to know that I am not alone and that others do care and can help if I let them. I am never alone when I let God help.

"Stop Smoking Tips: When you feel that you may smoke, think about the '5 Ds': 1) Do something else. Stop thinking about a cigarette and get up and do something… take a walk, read the Bible, or call someone on the telephone. 2) Drink lots of water… water is good for you and it cleans out your body. 3) Delay for five minutes… everyone can control themselves for a few minutes. Time yourself when the urge hits, before you know it the urge has passed. 4) Do deep, slow breathing to make it through urges or stressful times. 5) Do not smoke. Tell yourself you can make it through without that cigarette."

Readings: Psalms 23: "The Lord is my shepherd; I shall not want. He maketh me to lie down in green pastures; he leadeth me beside the still waters. He restoreth my soul; he leadeth me in the paths of righteousness for His name's sake. Yea, though I walk through the valley of the shadow of death, I will fear no evil: for thou are with me; thy rod and they staff they comfort me. Thou prepares a table before me in the presence of mine enemies; thou anointed my head with oil; my cup runneth over. Surely goodness and mercy shall follow me all the days of my life: and I will dwell in the house of the Lord forever." Psalms 119:144: "The righteous of thy testimonies is everlasting, Give me understanding, and I shall live." Job 28:28: "And to man He said, Behold the fear of the Lord, that is wisdom, and to depart from evil is understanding."

Taped Messages

Cassette tapes are another simple way of getting the word out. Many churches tape Sunday sermons, so there is always the opportunity for mass distribution of a sermon on a health topic. Give away the tapes or set up a pass-it-along tape ministry to allow even more people to hear the important message about health. Provide the tapes to other churches and organizations for playing at meetings or for individual members of the congregation to use.

Spiritual and Devotional Guides

An example of the innovative strategies that churches can use is the 30-day spiritual guide to stopping smoking, developed by Project BLESS, Baltimore Leading Everyone to Stop Smoking, a collaborative effort between the Clergy United for the Renewal of East Baltimore and the Johns Hopkins Center for Health Promotion. The guide, "PROJECT BLESS, Quit, For God... For Good!," was a 4-x-5 flip chart that resembled a small gift calendar, and provided motivation and encouragement to carry out a self-administered program through daily information, directives, and scriptural references. Here are a few of its daily messages:

Day 1. Think of your reasons to quit and write them down. This is something you have to do. Quitting smoking is something that everyone can do. The Lord smiles kindly on those who take the first steps toward healing! He will help prepare you for that glorious day when you will be rid of a costly and harmful habit. Take that first step. Think about getting cigarettes out of your life. Make a list of your reasons to quit smoking.
Psalms 37:23 The steps of a good man are ordered by the Lord; and he delighteth in his way.

Day 4. Realize that nicotine is a powerful drug. If you are afraid to let go of your cigarettes, realize that your faith in the Lord can free you from the bondage of the nicotine habit. Faith will see you through and guide your way. Millions of people quit smoking every year and you can too. Ask the Lord for help to break free.
Psalms 28:1 The Lord is my light and my salvation; who shall I fear? The Lord is the strength of my life; of whom shall I be afraid?

Day 6. Children who are around smokers get sick more often. Quitting smoking will clean the body, restore the mind and cure the spirit. Smoking not only harms you, but harms others especially our beloved children. By quitting, you can help children who are dear to you.
2 Corinthians 7:1 Having therefore these promises, dearly beloved, let

us cleanse ourselves from all filthiness of flesh and sprit, perfecting holiness in the fear of God.

Day 10. If you continue to smoke, you will reap only pain and suffering. Cigarettes provide only temporary satisfaction. Quit smoking and learn that God can give you complete satisfaction forever and ever. Prepare a plan of how you will quit. Let the Lord show you the way. *Psalms 51:10 Create in me a clean heart, O God; and renew a right spirit within me.*

Day 17. Be proud of yourself and let go of negative thoughts. The Lord will give you strength to quit smoking. Know that you are God's creation and worthy of his blessing. By stopping smoking you will be doing something wonderful. Let go of any negative thoughts you have about yourself. Be proud and know God loves you.
Jeremiah 17:14 Heal me, O Lord, and I shall be healed; save me, and I shall be saved: for thou art my praise.

Day 21. Throw out all your cigarettes. Put away old mistakes. Start anew. Clean your clothes and house. Get rid of all ashtrays. The Temple of the Lord is a holy place. Begin again with a pure heart. To stay smoke free, do not buy any cigarettes.
1 Corinthians 6:19-20 What? Know ye not that your body is the temple of the Holy Ghost which is in you, which ye have a God, and ye are not your own. For ye are bought with a price; therefore glorify God in your body, and in your spirit, which are God's.

Day 26. Keep busy to avoid smoking. When tempted to smoke, remember that smoking will not solve any problems... it just gives you one more thing to feel bad about. If you ask, the Lord will teach you to take one day at a time. To keep from smoking, keep your hands and mind busy. Just tell yourself to do something else instead of smoking. *Ecclesiastes 9:10 Whatsoever thy hand findeth to do, do it with thy might; for there is no work, nor device, nor knowledge, nor wisdom in the grave, wither thou goest.*

Day 29. Stay smoke free. Cigarettes had control over you and they can take control again if you get overconfident. Don't test yourself by smoking a cigarette. The only way to be smoke-free is to never smoke even one cigarette. God does not want you to fail. You must trust in God and abide in Him for full recovery. Enjoy being free at last. With God's help you can stay smoke-free.

John 15:7, 11 If ye abide in me, and my words abide in you, ye shall ask what ye will and it shall be done unto you. These things I have spoken unto you, that my joy might remain in you, and that your joy might be full.

This approach can also be used for other personal health programs. The Light Way Project is based out of the Center for Health Promotion at The Johns Hopkins School of Medicine. This weight loss and nutrition project to reduce heart disease produced a day-by-day devotional guide to help people measure and reduce their daily fat intake. *Day by Day, The Light Way! 28 Days of Inspirational Messages* featured a fat counter that listed foods and the calories and fats of particular portions. Categories included beverages, breads and cereals, dairy products, desserts, fast foods, oils and fats, frozen entrees, meats, chicken and other poultry, seafood, soups and sauces, and vegetables and fruit. The devotional guide consisted of 28 days of inspirational messages, scriptures, and an activity that supported the devotion of the day. As examples:

Day 8 Try It.

Please test your servants to 10 days, and let them give us vegetables to eat and water to drink, Daniel 1:12.

By trying something for a short period of time you will find that you can do it for a long time. Just as God showed Daniel and his friends how to be healthy, He wants us to be healthy. Change does not come overnight, but we must press on to a higher goal. You will soon find that you will feel better and are able to make healthy eating a habit. What I Can Do: For the coming week, try eating a double portion of vegetables and a smaller portion of meat. You will notice in the fat-counter tables that vegetables are low in fat, especially compared with most meats.

Day 10 Temperance.
And everyone who competes for the prize is temperate in all things, I Corinthians 9:25.

Eating healthily does not mean cutting out high-fat foods all the time. It is how often and how much you eat that is important. What I Can Do: For those few times when you must eat high-fat foods, here are some things you can do to lower how much fat you eat. Note those things you can try to do the next time you eat a high-fat food: have one piece of fried chicken instead of two, have one scoop of ice cream instead of two, eat a small piece of cake rather than a large one, order a hamburger without the cheese, sauce, or bacon.

Day 15 Self-Indulgence.
Woe to you Scribes and Pharisees, hypocrites. For you cleanse the outside of the cup and dish, but within you are full of exhortation and self-indulgence, Matthew 23:25.

God, our creator, knows the nature of our hearts. Do you outwardly give the impression that you are living a healthy life, but in private continue in bad habits? The Lord is ready to help you make changes in your life so that you can be clean and healthy on the inside as well as the outside. What I Can Do: The first step in reducing fat intake is learning where fat comes from. Today, read a food label and write down the name of the food and how many grams of fat is in one serving. Is this the type of information you could place on the bulletin board, hand out, or include in the church bulletin?

To get some consistent yet personalized messages delivered at a reduced cost, a group of ministers produced and distributed a guidebook that they adapted to each participating church but retained the same content for all versions. The messages in these booklets were prepared to reflect what the reader may be actually thinking, feeling, and experiencing. Maybe there are some members of your congregations who would be willing to share how they felt while experiencing a particular health problem? Consider public testimonies, poems, plays, and written testimonies such as the ones below:

When Life is Hard

People pushing and fighting and clouding my mind, Lord for your sake, won't you help me to take one day at a time.

When life gets hard because of family problems, money worries, concerns about work and children, I may tell myself that maybe now is not the time to quit smoking.

Smoking is the only way of dealing with my troubles—so why fight it. When I am tempted to smoke, I must remember that smoking will not solve any problems, it just gives me one more thing to feel bad about.

Everyone goes through hard times. Smokers use nicotine, a drug, to get through these bad times. People use drugs because it is a fast and an easy way to feel better. The drug may make me think I am being helped. Cigarettes are not my friends. They are really my enemy. To get through bad times I need to turn for support to the Lord, not to drugs like cigarettes.

Cigarettes never solve problems. I am lying to myself why I use cigarettes to deal with my problems. Through prayer and quiet thought I can find the strength to fight off my desire for cigarettes.

Health Fairs

Do you look around your community and think about good locations to set up health screenings? To be effective, you often have to take the service to the community. Rather than waiting for people to come to them, one organization went out and marketed its availability to conduct health fairs. The thrust of the group's message was that they could conduct health fairs virtually anywhere and at any location. A simple, one-panel flyer encouraged groups to plan and participate in health fairs that they planned in their communities. The East Baltimore Heart, Body, and Soul Project focused on preventing heart disease and strokes by offering free health fairs to community groups, churches, community centers, pharmacies, and grocery stores. They welcomed the involvement of groups in planning and participating in the health fairs, offering cholesterol, diabetes, and blood pressure tests; counseling to stop smoking; and counseling from a nurse, nutritionist, or health educator about the results of tests. When they identified health problems, they provided guidance for finding further care.

Is food prepared at your church? Has anyone ever examined the nutritional value of the food served? Can you include recipes in your church newsletter? Think about a church cookbook. Overall, think about ways to share healthy cooking and eating within and outside the church. One group used a health fair as an opportunity to share healthy eating information by incorporating a "health food fest" to promote healthy living. The Community Health Festival, held in Nashville, Tennessee, was cosponsored by several churches and local businesses and took place at the Corinthian Baptist Church. The organizers printed a booklet that included: cold and hot menu card recipes for clipping, herbal combinations for seasonings, lists of vegetables and meats known for healing qualities, simple foods that provide medical relief from illnesses, and warnings about foods proven to increase the risk of certain diseases. The recipes included fruit punch, chicken vegetable salad, oven fried chicken, grilled spicy chicken breast fillets, lemon-baked chicken, carrot and raisin salad, tossed salad with low-fat dressing, green beans, whole wheat rolls, bread and crackers, "lite" dairy topping, fresh strawberries, and angel food cake. Two sample dishes included in the booklet follow:

Oven Fried Chicken (serves 4)

Ingredients: Vegetable oil spray; one 2 1/2-3 lb. frying chicken, cut into serving pieces, skinned, with all visible fat removed; 1 cup skim milk; 1 cup cornflake crumbs; 1 teaspoon rosemary; and 2 teaspoons freshly ground black pepper.

Preparation: Preheat the oven to 400° F. Line a baking pan with foil and lightly spray it with vegetable oil. Rinse the chicken and pat it dry. Set the chicken aside. Pour milk into a shallow bowl. Combine the cornflake crumbs, rosemary, and pepper in another shallow bowl. Dip the chicken first into milk and then into the crumb mixture. Allow the chicken to stand briefly so the coating will adhere. Arrange the chicken in the prepared pan so pieces do not touch. Bake for 45 minutes or until done. The crumbs will form a crisp skin.

Nutrient Analysis: Calories 246 kcal, Cholesterol 93mg, Saturated Fat 2gm, Sodium 183 mg, Total Fat 7gm, Polyunsaturated Fat 2gm, Monounsaturated Fat 2gm.

Green Beans *(serves 8)*

Ingredients: 1 lb. of fresh green beans, rinsed and trimmed, or a 16-oz. can unsalted Italian green beans; 2 cups canned unsalted tomatoes; 1/2 cup of chopped celery; 1/4 cup of chopped green bell pepper; and 1/2 teaspoon onion powder.

Preparation: Cook the green beans until tender and then drain them. In a skillet, combine the green beans, tomatoes, celery, bell pepper, and onion powder. Cook over medium heat 15 minutes or until thoroughly heated.

Nutrient Analysis: Calories 26 kcal, Cholesterol 0mg, Saturated Fat 0gm, Sodium 18 mg, Total Fat 0gm, Polyunsaturated Fat 0gm, Monounsaturated Fat 0gm.

As these examples clearly show, there are many ways to incorporate the message of healthy living through church-related marketing, public relations, and communications. The key is to recognize all of the opportunities and act upon them as they become available, or create some special or unique opportunities of your own that are appropriate for the audience. Communication methods may change, but the real change occurs when a life has been saved or the quality of life is improved by something as simple as putting health tips on paper fans or outdoor church signs that normally list service times.

In most inner-city and community-based efforts, the more grassroots your marketing efforts are, the more effective the results. Don't hesitate to try new and different strategies, but keep in mind that they may not be effective if they are too high-tech or complicated.

Note: Information on programs in this chapter is from the following publications and organizations: *One Day at A Time, For Personal Guidance in Quitting Smoking,* the Clergy United for Renewal of East Baltimore, 1991; *Day by Day, The Light Way! 28 Days of Inspirational Messages* by the ministers of Heart, Body, and Soul; Project BLESS, *Quit, for God ... For Good,* Clergy United for the Renewal of East Baltimore and the Johns Hopkins Center for Health Promotion, 1993; Corinthian Baptist Church Health Festival Program, Nashville, Tennessee, September 23, 1995; and the East Baltimore Heart, Body, and Soul Project.

CHAPTER SIX

Profile of a Program and Partnership

THIS SUMMARY OF A SUCCESSFUL PROGRAM and partnership is just one example of how collaborations can make a difference. This program took place in East Baltimore, Maryland, a primarily African American community with more than its share of medical and social ills. The community of roughly 150,000, with approximately two churches on every city block, ranks among the highest in excess and premature morbidity and mortality in Maryland and in the United States. The overall mortality rates here and those from diabetes, strokes, and heart disease are greater than state or national rates. Premature deaths and disability from chronic and infectious diseases are very high, reflecting the high incidence of AIDS, asthma, cancer, high blood pressure, obesity, tuberculosis, and other illnesses. In addition, crime and substance abuse have taken a toll on the quality of life in the community. Approximately 20 percent of the population is on medical assistance and one third lives below the poverty level. Compared to the total population of the United States, this high-risk population had higher hospitalizations, urgent care treatment, and emergency room visits because preventative and health maintenance methods were nonexistent or underutilized. Traditional approaches to turn the tide on the health and social conditions simply did not work. These approaches tend to isolate health issues from social issues. Both have to be addressed for success. As the following profile demonstrates, the future of healthy communities lies in active partnerships among community and academic and professional colleagues. Further, I believe that similar programs involving the church will benefit the community and the research team equally.

Heart, Body, and Soul

Heart, Body, and Soul was formed as a proactive partnership to address the needs of the community, combining the strengths of the Johns Hopkins Academic Health Center and the community organization Clergy for the Renewal of East Baltimore (CURE), along with the Baltimore City Health Department, Baltimore City School System, and Health Care for the Homeless. Key to the group's success was that everyone was an equal partner, no one dominated as each contributed unique skills. The primary, and essential, parts of this partnership were community-based leadership, community ownership of programs, training and utilization of community residents, joint planning, cultural sensitivity training, training for students and faculty, evaluation strategies, long-term relationship planning, and community-based health care promotions.

As discussed in earlier chapters, there were several important lessons for the institution to learn about the community, particularly that African Americans are not all alike. Even within the same community, there are cultural differences and preferences and a range of personalities and classes. Equally important were the observations and adjustments that the church and institution had to make to work together to develop a central mission statement. It is a useful example of a community-based public health initiative mission statement, listing specific goals and actions.

As a community in East Baltimore incorporating residents, the health and educational institutions of Baltimore City, the Johns Hopkins University, and organizations serving East Baltimore, our united purpose is to promote the health and social well-being of East Baltimore with the ultimate goal of improving the health status of the community.

We do this by: (1) Creating enduring partnerships between the East Baltimore community, educational institutions, and health and human services organizations. (2) Developing, implementing and evaluating a community-based public health model that will enhance training, policy, education, and service programs. (3) Planning to sustain and disseminate the successful elements of the community-based public health model throughout the city and state. (4) Collecting process and outcome-based data to demonstrate, where possible, improved health status of individuals and the community. (5) Linking issues of health to issues of poverty, hopelessness, and social and economic conditions.

In forming the partnership, a solid commitment was made to the following principles: (1) Realization that the community is already "in power" rather than being "empowered," owning the decision-making process and not just serving as a participant or informant. (2) Avoiding the "rescue fantasy" or "handout" mentality. (3) Working to establish mutual respect and trust among partners. (4) Aiming for diversity at all levels, including leadership. (5) Agreeing to disagree and recognize different values, yet at the same time adopting one common vision. (6) Streamlining planning and minimizing red tape. Accepting being part of an evolutionary paradigm. Being flexible but malleable. (7) Accepting that there will be personal and professional risks. (8) Never giving up.

Further, the group identified considerations for institutions seeking to establish successful programs in African American communities: (1) Take time to understand the community overall as it has a different history, based on its heritage and an ongoing struggle to survive. (2) Remember that there is a spiritual side. With technology advances it is easy to forget that you are dealing with a spiritual group of people. (3) Recognize that agencies and institutions and their representatives are foreigners in the community. Don't expect the community to adapt to your ways, see how you can adapt to the ways of the community. (4) Be patient, understanding that members of the community have had a long, hard journey. Brief contact should not be expected to produce immediate or huge results. (5) Show a genuine interest in the way the community operates by attending functions, listening, and seeking help in understanding. (6) Don't simply seek the advice of the community, but include the community by developing a team relationship, especially with community leaders. (7) Understand that the natural communications network of the community is that of residents talking to each other rather than relying upon the written word. Therefore, don't depend solely on the written word to get information out. (8) These communities belong to the residents, they have power and do not need empowering. If the program is to last, you must accept that the community must eventually own it because when you are gone, the residents will still be in the community and some of the problems will remain. (9) Don't assume that all of the residents are alike. Inner-city communities are rich with diversity, with doctors, lawyers, teachers, traditional and non-traditional families, and others, just like mainstream society. Not everyone is illiterate, unemployed, uninsured, or uninterested in their health status. The diversity and culture of the community must be recognized together.

One of Heart, Body, and Soul's first projects was to test strategies to reduce the number of cigarette smokers among East Baltimore African Americans. (This particular intervention project was funded by the National Institutes of Health, National Heart, Lung, and Blood Institute Grant, RO1 HL 4360, "Church-based Smoking Cessation Strategies in an Urban Black Community.") Specifically, the goal was to increase smoking-cessation rates among church attendees. Although churches, with their strong volunteer orientation and information sharing network, are an excellent source for reaching people, many individuals are often embarrassed about their smoking behavior, may not want to participate publicly, or may not want to reveal their need for help. However, those who did come forward were very active participants and less comfortable with a public pronouncement of their smoking problem still benefited from the sermons, testimonies, and printed materials. It is likely that these individuals may participate in future activities or may attempt to cut back or stop smoking independently. Thus, multiple messages and opportunities to learn about the dangers of smoking are most beneficial.

Other published smoking-cessation strategies targeted to African Americans have often had little to no effect because the efforts were based on models tested and used with majority white populations. The HBS project was a culture-sensitive approach that targeted church attendees. Out of 130 churches in the area, 22 of different denominations were recruited. Twenty-nine lay volunteers were trained as smoking-cessation specialists to implement intervention activities at churches and an additional 272 church members conducted health screenings at their own churches. Clergy United for the Renewal of East Baltimore served as the primary agency representing local clergy for the project. The entire process—recruitment, planning, communications, training, and evaluation—of this innovative approach was one that was challenging on both ends as it required compromise, changing of perceptions, and a willingness to accept that some differences will always remain. Out of this has come a systematic approach that has proven to be effective not only for the smoking-cessation program but also for combating heart disease, diabetes, asthma, and other illnesses.

Although pastors did not initially identify smoking as a top-priority concern among the church and community, once the statistics for the city and community were revealed the clergy realized the major impact of smoking-related morbidity and mortality. African Americans smoke cigarettes at rates higher than whites, with alarmingly high rates among women. Further, previous smoking-cessation strategies targeted and implemented for African Americans had low success rates, attributed to trying to use the same strategies for majority and minority populations. Thus, it was important to develop a culturally sensitive approach involving the pastors of the church at practically every level and to incorporate spiritual as well as cultural sensitivities into the project from its beginning. The pastors were the only persons who could bring this very important element to the project.

First, an advisory committee meeting was held between representatives from the churches, public sector, voluntary organizations, and local health and social and human service agencies. At this one-time gathering, the president of CURE became the official leader, without any monetary compensation or support, to coordinate the churches' involvement. Next, a leadership and development structure had to be put in place. In doing so, it was important to make sure that the individuals involved had no self-promotion objectives and could focus strictly on the project. Secondly, the group needed to be diverse to represent appropriately the population to be served; in this case, church members from different denominations. It was important to make it clear that the work was strictly voluntary, with no promises or plans for future compensation, employment, or favors of any kind. Legal bylaws were needed to ensure the proper functioning of the group, decision-making procedures, obligations and expectations, and other rules to build a strong and sound organization. From there, a Heart, Body, and Soul Steering Committee of three pastors from different denominations was recruited to work with the institution's investigators and 22 participating churches. The Steering Committee met routinely, usually bimonthly during the first year, and the president of CURE frequently attended these meetings as well. Because the Steering Committee had a general mistrust of outside institutions, the initial meetings focused on fleshing out ownership and control issues, developing the working relationship, and discussing planning and implementation. With final approval resting with CURE, the Steering Committee selected the project's title, logo, and mission statement, and handled the hiring of project staff. It also advised and was involved in the development of intervention strategies, operational aspects, research design, and data collection.

An issue often underestimated by those hoping to work with churches is that all churches do not function alike. Although the pastor may have agreed to participate, the acceptance of Heart, Body, and Soul and the ease of its implementation varied from church to church, depending upon the size and demographics of the congregation, the level of support for the pastor and his length of tenure, other active or attempted health ministries, and the congregation's pattern of internal versus external outreach programs. These were factors that both parties learned to consider, once the Steering Committee began to work.

While some information was known about the community, a comprehensive needs assessment of the residents of the community was conducted through the use of surveys, individualized approaches, focus groups, and observations. The actual catchment area covered 21 census tracts in East Baltimore with a population in 1992 of 71,292 people, of whom 47,438 were African American males over 21 years of age. The total unemployment rate among eligible workers was about one third, 68 percent had lived in the same house for five years or more and belonged to a community church, 57 percent had a high school diploma, and 46 percent had annual incomes below the poverty level. The project area was determined through block observations of areas within the community with churches, commercial establishments, schools, recreation centers, libraries, and community, health, human service, and social service organizations. The steering committee visited churches, attended events, made contacts with city and state elected officials, and investigated smoking ordinances and legislation.

Through these efforts, a social map was developed that also identified the influences in the community and the components of the map were verified through a communitywide telephone survey. This survey was able to indicate the prevalence of smoking among the African American population relevant to such factors as age, gender, and education. It also revealed what influenced residents to smoke, perceptions of health risks, environmental factors, and reaction to the pressure to quit. The findings from this random-digit dialing survey were compared with the data collected through the churches and community research. The survey concluded with 941 interviews. While the information received was wider in scope than originally planned, it was still very valuable. For example, it revealed that self-reported smoking was higher than rates reported by a 1987 Behavioral Risk Factor Survey; the number of former smokers was very low; more than 55 percent stated that they attended church regularly, with at least 31 percent attending occasionally; and 98 percent indicated that religion was an important aspect of their life, with 82 percent listening to religious or gospel music. To further confirm the findings, focus groups were conducted among 31 current and former smokers during three sessions. Participants were recruited from church health fairs and provided many insights that became critical to the implementation of the project. Some of these were: (1) Restricting smoking in public areas influenced smoking behavior strongly. (2) There was a high level of knowledge of smoking health risks and exposure to antismoking methods. (3) Cold turkey was the most often used method for quitting. (4) Children and support from God or the church were motivational factors in quitting, not support from family or friends. (5) Nicotine replacement therapy was viewed as substituting one addiction for another and was rejected by the majority of the participants.

Once the participating churches had been identified and some basic research had been conducted, the next step was to orient the church leadership to the project. This orientation process included face-to-face meetings, which were difficult to arrange because of the busy schedule of pastors. The meetings focused on an overview of the project and the level of the pastor's interest in promoting health issues among the congregation. The Heart, Body, and Soul Smoking Cessation Program was identified as the first vehicle to introduce a health initiative at the church. Upon agreeing, the pastor and church entered into a covenant that detailed the roles of the congregation and the project. Eleven of the participating churches were randomly selected for minimal intervention strategies to decrease smoking. These churches did not receive training, group support sessions, or pastoral sermons. Pastors were aware of the random selection process but were generally not concerned, as minimal intervention sites would still have health fairs and access and attention to smoking data and smoking issues, such as copies of American Lung Association pamphlets for distribution. The remaining 21 churches had intensive intervention activities. To begin, baseline health screenings and assessments were conducted at churches on high-attendance days. After churchwide mobilization events and training sessions, a special

Sunday kick-off service was held and promotional materials were distributed. These materials included customized fact sheets, a book of devotions to assist smokers, and a stop-smoking inspirational tape. Announcements, material distribution, testimonies and other awareness and recruitment activities took place over the next three weeks.

The actual health screenings were scheduled to meet the specific requirements of the people administering the program, the church, and its congregation. A total of 1,290 church members were screened and received risk-reduction counseling. Trained volunteers and church nurses organized and conducted the health screenings. They then recruited church members to participate in a two-hour health fair training session that was primarily participatory and hands-on in nature. The training format included an orientation to the organization and project, the role of the volunteer(s), work standards, community resource mapping, community organizing, a perspective on community health prevention and promotion, goal setting, care planning, documentation, and outreach conduct. A curriculum was designed for the training and for conducting screening and intervention activities. Some of the specific topics covered were, "How to Hold a Prepare to Quit Session," "How to Hold a Spiritual Support Session," "Encouragement for Smokers," and "Encouragement for Cessation Specialists." The amount of time spent on these and other issues varied based upon knowledge and skills and comfort level of the individuals in training. Of note is that many of the participants were nursing assistants, LPNs, and RNs. At least 230 adults and 42 teenagers were trained during four or more sessions.

One church was identified as a model for the intensive intervention strategy, and the pastor of this lead church and all others involved assisted with planning and conducting the interventions. To incorporate the spiritual aspect, the intensive intervention model included devotional books, prayer, testimonials, group support sessions led by trained lay volunteers, sermons, gospel music, and audiotapes. Every effort was made to utilize the actual church site for activities to enhance church ownership of the project, to have access to the church members, and to sustain the project's efforts. At least three weeks were spent in preparing the church congregation for the upcoming program and then another three weeks were spent on active church intervention activities. Group support continued for another four weeks or more.

To reinforce the program, during church the pastors recognized all smoking-cessation activities and distributed certificates of merit for up to six months after the program was implemented. Three of the churches began to offer regular support groups, continuing the testimonies and the sermons beyond the initial phase, some for up to a year or more. Twenty-one of the churches agreed to have follow-up health fairs at the one-year benchmark and 91 percent of the participants were reinterviewed by telephone, home visits, or at health fairs. Ongoing smoking-cessation program data were collected using exhaled carbon monoxide and other tests.

The development and implementation period for the smoking-cessation program spanned from 1 to 11 months. Three months were spent on the formation of the Steering Committee and the community resource inventory. Both the baseline telephone survey and follow-up smoker interviews required four months of work for completion. Church recruitment, mobilization, and meetings at the 22 sites totaled five months of effort. Developing support materials that were generic but could be customized took six months, while follow-up health fairs required eight months of work. The formation of the Advisory Committee and implementation of the minimal intervention strategy required about one month of work each. The two longest periods of work were the nine months for the baseline health fairs, including volunteer recruitment, training, and smoker interviews, and the intensive intervention activities, which lasted 11 months.

The partnership not only affected the health status and consciousness of a segment of the inner-city population in East Baltimore, it also changed how institutions and community organizations felt about their abilities to work together. Questions were asked to gauge their mutual perceptions of one another. Of particular interest was any change in the historical ill-will towards Johns Hopkins University, including community-wide beliefs that human experimentation and surveys were often conducted with no real benefit to the community. In the past, researchers would come into the community, conduct their studies, and leave nothing behind. While this was not the case with Heart, Body, and Soul, these types of attitudes and experiences had to be addressed before they created a climate of distrust and anger that could have jeopardized this partnership and program.

The partners agreed that the alliance created a valuable forum for communication and interaction that could serve as a model for other organizations and a wider population base. While Heart, Body, and Soul led to an improvement in the relationship between the community and the institution, it was among a limited segment. Greater trust will have to come from additional programs that reach broader segments. The group also recognized that there was a need to get more women involved in the project, from administration to treatment. The barriers here were the lack of transportation for the elderly, child care availability, accessible locations, and the need for more flexible hours and days. One issue that surfaced was a major disparity between what the community expected from such a large organization and what the organization could actually provide. Some thought that the community expectations were unrealistic, while others felt that the institution was holding back. These feelings changed somewhat with an improved understanding of the other's circumstances, policies, restrictions, needs, and resources. Another finding was that the community believed that the institution was dragging its feet. Actually, this perception derives from a community culture and people accustomed to immediate action over the often long and drawn-out efforts of well-intentioned projects because of institutional structure, checks and balances, priorities, and numerous other projects. These somewhat unchangeable factors were viewed as a lack of genuine interest, but contact and interaction at the community level helped bring about a better understanding of how institutions operate.

On a larger, more national scale several considerations were presented for examination and possible implementation. Most of these suggestions were targeted at the federal, state, and local levels, including the private sector. It was felt that these types of incentives would be necessary to truly affect the complexity and sheer magnitude of the needs of those in the inner cities. These included: (1) A commitment of academic institutions to partnering with surrounding communities that address not only health issues, but related social, economic, and environmental situations. (2) A greater commitment to increase education among students and faculty relative to community-based services, along with including real experience. (3) The possibility of federal grant funding for academic institutions partnering with communities that are in need and underserved. (4) Incentives, through grants, matching funds, and low-interest loans, for communities to create neighborhood health centers. (5) Funds for both health professionals and community health workers to provide services in the areas of disease prevention and health promotion. (6) Tax benefits for businesses and financial institutions that provide support and loans to community and academic alliances. (7) Regulation and monitoring of primary care practices. (8) Certification of a new health care "paraprofessional" at the community level. (9) Formal recognition of churches and community organizations as an important complement to traditional health care.

In summary, attitudes toward the partnership improved more among the alliance than the larger community. There was tremendous enthusiasm in the progress made, but a nagging reminder that still more needs to be done before coming close to mutual understanding and complete trust. What is probably most important is that now there is at least one formula to use again and again with potential spin-off programs for additional collaborative efforts. Not to be lost or forgotten, though, are all of the people who benefited through training and health services, including the church leaders, congregations, institution leaders, teachers, students, and community health workers.

In the long run, everyone realized that all were better off working together than remaining apart.

CHAPTER SEVEN

From the Pulpit and the People

THIS CHAPTER PRESENTS SEVERAL WAYS that health information can be shared with church congregations, how community residents have benefited, and what students and teachers have learned. Songs and sermons about good health, as these examples show, can reach deep inside the community, touch those unable to attend church, and spread outside the church and through the community. Further on in the chapter, you will read actual testimonials and stories from people who responded to the message to improve health care and who took advantage of what a partnership can offer a community.

The Gospel of Good Health

Many ministers who participate in community-based public health projects take advantage of the opportunity to stress the importance of good health habits to their congregations during songs and sermons. These songs and sermons are part of the church service, seen on television, heard on the radio or tapes, and viewed on video. In Baltimore, Pastor James Carter and the Little Ark Missionary Baptist Church developed a song to inspire smoking cessation:

Solo Female: Life is so short, but it is oh so sweet,
and we all have problems that we must meet,
The habits we have seem so hard to break,
all because we want to do it our way.
Smoke cigarettes but say no to drugs,
they both are the same and do destroy.

Our loved ones pass on and children are born
continuing the habit of the nicotine drug.

Chorus: So let's pull together and help one another,
smoking can bring sufferin', pain and trouble.
Millions of people die each day,
all because of a habit hard to break.

Solo: In God we find strength, so let him control
our hearts and our habits and our souls.
And, if you think you can do it alone,
then you'll face a long, lonely road.

Chorus   So let's pull together and help one another
and Soloist: smoking can bring sufferin', pain and trouble.
Millions of people die each day,
all because of a habit hard to break.
So let's pull together and help one another
smoking can bring sufferin', pain and trouble.
Millions of people die each day.
all because of a habit hard to break
all because of a habit hard to break
all because of a habit hard to break.

For those of you who are ministers, several sermons follow that
you may want to use as a reference as you prepare your own. If you
are not a minister, these sermons will give you an idea of how information regarding health can be delivered from the minister directly
to however many people attend services. That number can range
from less than 100 to 3,000 or more, even before factoring in the
people who will hear about the sermon later. It is common for

someone in the community to ask another, "How was the sermon today?," "What did the preacher preach about?," or "What was the message today?" The following is an original sermon by the Reverend Dr. Melvin B. Tuggle II.

It's in my Heart (Cleaning up our Hearts)

The heart is deceitful above all things and desperately wicked. Who can know it? The Bible mentions at least 50 types of hearts. There is the troubled heart, heavy heart, hard heart, single heart, foolish heart, true heart, broken heart, willing heart, proud heart, wicked heart, pure heart, and unsearchable heart, just to name a few. The word heart is listed in the scriptures at least 821 times. When we study the scriptures, we learn that the word "heart" is used in various ways.

There are six distinct ways that the word heart is used and it is time for "good old" churchfolk to stop the sin of smoking. Smoking causes physical heart disease. We need to clean our hearts. Let me share some important information about the physical heart and why we need to clean it up. The number one killer among African Americans is heart disease and that includes strokes, high cholesterol, high blood pressure, and heart attacks. It may surprise some of you that crack, AIDS, sickle cell, cancer, and genocide are not the number one killers among us. Instead, heart disease is the number one killer.

We need to clean our hearts because this old ticker pumps more than a million quarts of blood in a lifetime. We must be watchful because neglect of our physical hearts will send us to an early grave. The physical heart needs to be clean. Medical experts tell us that smoking is a leading contributor to heart disease; yet, some of us continue to light up and puff away. Many of us have cheated God of our service because we neglected our health. But, now is the time for "good old" Christians to clean our hearts. Every time a Christian man, woman, boy, or young woman puffs on a cigarette they are filling their heart with poison. It is time for God's children to take to heart that they can do all things through Christ who strengthens them. The heart is deceitful and desperately wicked and because of that we need God to search and research our hearts. Then, we need to call upon Him to rid of us our dangerous addiction to nicotine. (Reference: Jeremiah 17:9.)

The Community Responds

Margaret Matthews was not an expert about her diabetes, but she knew she had to "keep a check on it." For years, she depended on hospital clinics to do just that. "Then the clinic closed," she recalls. "I was just petrified. I felt lost, with nowhere to go. I thought it was terrible." She then heard about the Oliver Prevention Center in East Baltimore, which is supported by the Community-Based Public Health Initiative and run by Heart, Body, and Soul, a subsidiary of Clergy United for the Renewal of East Baltimore (CURE). "My friend was going there for a free cholesterol screening and invited me to go along," she says. Afterwards, Matthews received a letter informing her about a diabetes education class. "I said certainly, I would go." And she did. The comprehensive diabetes program takes a week to complete, and includes a range of topics, from glucose testing and eye care to exercise and good nutrition. Qualified neighborhood health workers teach classes with an attendance rate of 90 percent among program participants. Because of growing demand, classes are now offered every other month rather than quarterly as before.

Matthews says the demand is high because "we all learned a lot about diabetes and how to manage it. They gave us free glucose machines to test our blood sugar levels. Many people in the class did not even know how to test their blood or what their blood sugar level should be. We had different speakers come in to tell us different things about diabetes. We learned so much." She wishes she had these classes years ago: "Going to the doctor may not be enough. They are not telling you about how diabetes affects your limbs, your body, or your eyesight. They just tell you they are putting you on insulin and you have to get your blood checked. You go back and they might say, well, you have to lose some weight or increase your insulin. My doctor had put me on some pills. I'd go home and eat whatever I wanted and take a pill. Nobody told me you have to eat a certain way. I did not have a machine and I was not checking my sugar every day. I just did not know. I did not know it was affecting the nerves in my feet, my circulation, and my eyesight. But, if you learn you can know what you are dealing with and you can live better. And, that is what I did not have until it was too late. I lost my leg."

When the classes were over, says Matthews, the classmates were hesitant to part company. "So we started a support group to keep in touch with each other. They made me the lead person. It has been wonderful. We meet once a month except in the summer. When people want to know different information, they will call me, or if somebody is having a problem, they will call me. If I can tell them something or help them, I do. If I feel down, I can call one of them. It is nice to talk to someone who really knows what you are going through. That can be a big help. Each person in the group has a buddy they can call and talk to anytime. I really do not know more than anyone else, but I put into practice what I have learned. I am doing well now because I know how to manage my diabetes and keep myself under control. I try to stress this to the rest of the group, that you have to take control of your diabetes. You cannot be like an ostrich and stick your head in a hole and hope the problem goes away, because it will not. When I was first diagnosed with diabetes, I weighed about 240 pounds. Now I am down to my ideal weight, I am not tired all the time, and I walk every day and keep busy. I do not want to see anyone go through what I went through. A lot of people do not know they have diabetes, and when they find out, they do not know what to do, or where to turn, or how to take care of themselves. That is why I am glad there are classes."

Joseph Swillings joined the Army when he was 18 and for the next eight years made a point of staying healthy and fit. After the Army, he worked as a laborer in a rock quarry until an accident in 1993 left him disabled. "Then my mother died, and my whole world turned upside down. I stopped taking care of myself. I just gave up," recalls Swillings. Then, one day he noticed the same center that Ms.

Matthews had visited, and wandered in to find out what was going on inside. "The health workers checked my blood pressure and said it was sky-high. They wanted me to go to Johns Hopkins. I already knew about the problem, and I did not care." But, by the summer of 1994 his kidneys failed.

He spent a month in the hospital and six months on dialysis. "I was taking minoxidil to control my pressure, but I had a reaction to the medicine. By February of 1995, there were two liters of fluid around my heart, and I went back into the hospital for a week." In August Swillings lost his worker's compensation benefits. "At that point, I had no medical assistance. A 10-day supply of the medicine I needed was $36.00. Roxie was one of the health workers who helped me at the Center. She got me a three-month supply of medicine and that saved me."

However, his problems were not over and the neighborhood health workers knew that was the case. They urged Swillings to go to the VA hospital for regular care but he was adamant about not going. He refused to consider the VA. "Back in 1985 I went to the VA hospital with a bad cold," he says. "They gave me such a run-around. Civilians can get very smart with you. They treated me so badly I said I would never, ever go back there." So Roxie and her colleagues, Christine and Teresa, worked on changing his mind. They counseled him and encouraged him, going as far as visiting his house to follow up if he did not come to the Center. "That impressed me. It made a big difference for me. There were things I could not talk to my family about, but I could tell the health workers because they were so caring," Swillings says. That caring finally created a change of heart. "It took 10 years and near death for me to go back to the VA, but they convinced me. I am off dialysis now and they have changed my medications five times to find the right one for me. My blood pressure is under control and I feel fine. I cannot praise the Center enough. Anybody who goes through those doors will be satisfied. The health workers are wonderful. I am 35 years old now and they made a big difference in my life. I will do anything to help the Center."

Teaching Health Workers and Students

Funding from the Kellogg Foundation was used to design an unusual course that combined unconventional teaching methods and unique learning opportunities. The course, Health and Homelessness, is offered twice a year and requires students to participate in two weekend seminars and complete a 10-week individual project on topics of value to those seeking to improve health care. Byron Hiebert-Crape, a doctoral student in epidemiology, describes Health and Homelessness as "one of those courses where you actually link with the community. I think it has really transformed many students, and I think it is absolutely necessary for all health students to take." Other course graduates think that all medical students should be required to take the course, along with local politicians.

"What makes this course unique," according to Hiebert-Crape, "is that so much of the teaching is from people in the community, including homeless people. How often do you have contact with the people you are learning about? It is not very often you can really come face-to-face with homeless people, and realize that they have insights—much more than you do about their situation. That is a rarity." The course is taught by staff at Health Care for the Homeless, a local, not-for-profit health care provider, and by homeless people who serve on panels. Students from various disciplines, even outside the health care field, and interested community residents take the course. They learn firsthand about the causes of homelessness, its health consequences, the barriers to care, and advocacy methods.

"It is an eye-opener and mind-opener for many, many students who may be well-read in homelessness, who might have compassion, or who might even have worked in a soup kitchen. To sit down and not only have these people tell you their stories, but sometimes to have them confront you to discuss issues that you have not an inkling about that involves their inner feelings and thoughts—that is something else. Or, to hear from others who work with the homeless every day and know them very well, that is unusual too. To have that kind of interaction is really challenging, because what changes your direction in life is human contact. That is when you start empathizing and feeling what another person is talking about. It is not an intellectual trip. When you start reaching down to something deeper, that is what changes people's lives," said Hiebert-Crape.

Mary Kate Heggarty, a first-year community health student, thought that of all the courses she took that year, the Health and Homelessness program made the greatest impression. "I had a preconceived notion of homelessness until I took this course," says Heggarty. "Two groups of homeless people spoke to us about their lives. It was not at all what I expected. Some were college graduates who had gotten involved in drugs. I will never forget that experience. You really cannot judge a book by its cover. Community nursing means seeing people in their own environment, understanding their circumstances, their perspectives, and their needs." Students in Hiebert-Crape's class had reactions similar to Heggarty's. As he describes it, "When you hear students' comments and questions in the beginning of the course, you realize how naive and far removed from reality many of them are at that point. They think maybe homeless people are just lazy. As they learn differently, many of them wind up working at shelters and other places in the city. I think their lives and careers will be very different because of the experience. Two students who recently took the class now want to study the impact of homelessness on children. They want to meet them and make contact with them. Once you do that, it is harder and harder to turn back." As one of the homeless men who served as a panelist, Andre Rhyme says, "We tell our stories, how we became homeless, and some of the things we went through being homeless, like our problems getting medical attention. A lot of the students are surprised, and afterward, many of them are compassionate. They feel more comfortable, and they make us feel more comfortable too. We trade information. When you have been on the streets, you learn about people very well. Some students come up to us and ask what they can do. I tell them one of the things you probably could do is to volunteer some of your time at a place like Health Care for the Homeless or some of the clinics in the city."

This type of interaction between students and the population that they may ultimately serve is invaluable. It allows for the real human contact that is critical to providing true public health services. There are so many ways to reach the community that require simply ingenuity and effort. Most important is to look for opportunities that are not common, but that may be particularly effective in reaching the targeted population. Do not be limited by what has been done before, within or outside your community. You will then be able to transfer that knowledge to the community health workers and others who have a stake in the survival of inner-city communities.

Index